OWEN HUNTER

Basal Cell Carcinoma

Your Comprehensive Blueprint for Diagnosis and Treatment

Contents

INTRODUCTION

Basal Cell Carcinoma: Unveiling the Complexities and Conquering the Challenge

In the vast landscape of dermatological conditions, few stand out as prominently as basal cell carcinoma (BCC). This insidious form of skin cancer, often characterized by its slow-growing yet persistent nature, has long been a subject of intense study and clinical concern. As one of the most commonly diagnosed cancers worldwide, BCC demands our unwavering attention and a comprehensive understanding of its multifaceted nature.

Affecting millions of individuals annually, basal cell carcinoma represents a significant public health burden. Its incidence continues to rise, driven by a complex interplay of environmental, genetic, and lifestyle factors. From sun exposure to inherited genetic predispositions, the underlying causes of BCC are diverse and often intertwined, posing a formidable challenge to healthcare providers and patients alike.

Yet, despite its prevalence, basal cell carcinoma has often been overshadowed by its more aggressive counterparts, such as melanoma. This misconception, however, is far from accurate. While BCC is rarely life-threatening when detected and treated early, its potential for local tissue destruction and disfigurement can have profound implications on an individual's quality of life. Neglecting the seriousness of this condition can lead to devastating consequences, both physically and psychologically.

In this comprehensive book, we delve deep into the intricate world of basal cell carcinoma, exploring its nuances, advancements in diagnostic techniques, and the ever-evolving landscape of treatment options. Our goal is to empower healthcare professionals, patients, and the general public with the knowledge and tools necessary to tackle this pervasive skin cancer effectively.

Understanding the Fundamentals of Basal Cell Carcinoma

At its core, basal cell carcinoma is a type of non-melanoma skin cancer that originates from the basal cells, the lowest layer of the epidermis. These cells are responsible for continuously replenishing the skin, ensuring its integrity and protective function. However, when genetic mutations or environmental factors disrupt this delicate balance, the basal cells can undergo uncontrolled proliferation, resulting in the formation of a BCC lesion.

Contrary to popular belief, basal cell carcinoma is not a single, homogeneous entity. It encompasses a diverse spectrum of subtypes, each with its own unique clinical characteristics and management considerations. From the most common nodular form to the more aggressive infiltrative and morpheaform variants, understanding the nuances of BCC subtypes is crucial for accurate diagnosis and tailored treatment approaches.

Moreover, the location of the BCC lesion can greatly influence the clinical presentation and the subsequent management strategy. Facial BCCs, for instance, may require more meticulous surgical planning to minimize scarring and preserve cosmetic and functional outcomes. Conversely, lesions on the trunk or extremities may pose different challenges, necessitating a balanced approach between oncological control and aesthetic considerations.

Navigating the Diagnostic Landscape

Accurate and timely diagnosis of basal cell carcinoma is the cornerstone of effective management. In this book, we delve into the comprehensive array of diagnostic tools available, empowering healthcare providers to make informed decisions and guide patients through the diagnostic process.

Visual examination and dermatoscopy have long been the mainstays of BCC diagnosis, enabling clinicians to identify characteristic features such as the presence of telangiectasias, translucent nodules, and the classic "pearly" appearance. However, advancements in imaging techniques, including high-frequency ultrasound and reflectance confocal microscopy, have enhanced our ability to visualize the depth and extent of BCC lesions, guiding treatment planning and improving patient outcomes.

The role of biopsy and histopathological analysis cannot be overstated. By obtaining a small sample of the suspicious lesion, healthcare providers can definitively confirm the diagnosis and gain valuable insights into the specific subtype of basal cell carcinoma. This information is crucial in developing a personalized treatment strategy, as different subtypes may require tailored approaches to achieve optimal results.

Empowering Patients through Early Detection and Prevention

In the realm of basal cell carcinoma, prevention and early detection are paramount. This book underscores the importance of skin self-examination, empowering patients to become active participants in their own healthcare. By recognizing the early signs of BCC and seeking timely medical attention, individuals can significantly improve their chances of successful treatment and minimize the risk of disease progression.

Moreover, the book delves into the vital role of primary care providers in the early detection and management of basal cell carcinoma. By incorporating routine skin examinations into standard practice and educating patients on risk factors, these healthcare professionals can play a pivotal role in identifying BCC lesions at their earliest stages, when treatment is most effective.

Screening and risk stratification strategies are also explored, highlighting the importance of identifying individuals with heightened susceptibility to BCC due to factors such as skin type, sun exposure history, and genetic predispositions. By targeting these high-risk populations, healthcare providers can implement tailored prevention and surveillance protocols, further enhancing early detection and improving patient outcomes.

Comprehensive Treatment Approaches

The management of basal cell carcinoma has evolved considerably over the years, with a repertoire of surgical and non-surgical treatment modalities available to healthcare providers. In this book, we delve into the intricacies of each approach, empowering readers to make informed decisions in collaboration with their healthcare team.

Surgical interventions, such as excision and Mohs micrographic surgery, remain the gold standard for the majority of BCC cases. By meticulously removing the tumor while preserving healthy tissue, these techniques offer excellent oncological control and favorable cosmetic outcomes. However, the book also explores alternative surgical options, including curettage, electrodessication, cryotherapy, and laser therapy, each with its unique advantages and indications.

For patients who may not be suitable candidates for surgery or those seeking non-invasive alternatives, this book highlights the role of topical medications, photodynamic therapy, and radiation therapy. These non-surgical approaches can be particularly beneficial for patients with multiple or recurrent BCC lesions, or for those located in challenging anatomical areas.

Importantly, the book also addresses the management of advanced and metastatic basal cell carcinoma, a rare but serious manifestation of the disease. Here, readers will find comprehensive insights into the use of targeted therapies, such as Hedgehog pathway inhibitors, and the emergence of combination treatment strategies that are revolutionizing the care of these complex cases.

Optimizing Outcomes and Quality of Life

Beyond the clinical aspects of basal cell carcinoma, this book places a strong emphasis on the patient-centered approach, addressing the multifaceted impact of this condition on an individual's well-being.

The chapter on cosmetic and functional outcomes underscores the importance of reconstruction techniques and the minimization of scarring and disfigurement. By recognizing the psychological and emotional toll that BCC can have on patients, the book equips healthcare providers with the knowledge and strategies to optimize aesthetic results and improve quality of life.

Equally crucial is the book's exploration of survivorship and long-term follow-up. Emphasizing the importance of meticulous recurrence monitoring and skin cancer prevention strategies, the book empowers patients to take an active role in their ongoing care, ensuring early detection and prompt intervention in the event of disease recurrence or the development of new lesions.

Furthermore, the book delves into the integration of complementary and alternative approaches, recognizing the growing interest in holistic wellness among patients. By examining the evidence-based efficacy of dietary modifications, stress management techniques, and other complementary therapies, the book provides a comprehensive framework for addressing the multifaceted needs of individuals with basal cell carcinoma.

Embracing Global Perspectives and Future Directions

In an increasingly interconnected world, this book acknowledges the global nature of basal cell carcinoma, exploring the variations in incidence, management strategies, and health disparities across different regions and populations. By examining the challenges faced by underserved communities and highlighting efforts to improve accessibility and affordability of care, the book aims to foster a more inclusive and equitable approach to BCC management.

Looking to the future, the book delves into the exciting realm of emerging technologies and research priorities. From innovative diagnostic tools and personalized treatment approaches to the exploration of novel therapeutic targets, readers will gain insights into the cutting edge of basal cell carcinoma care. This forward-looking perspective empowers healthcare professionals and patients alike to stay at the forefront of advancements in the field, ultimately improving patient outcomes and quality of life.

Conclusion

Basal cell carcinoma, though often perceived as a relatively benign skin cancer, demands our unwavering attention and a comprehensive understanding of its complexities. This book, designed to be a comprehensive and authoritative resource, aims to empower healthcare providers, patients, and the general public in the fight against this pervasive condition.

By delving into the intricacies of diagnosis, treatment, and patient-centered care, this book serves as a valuable tool for navigating the ever-evolving landscape of basal cell carcinoma management. Through the integration of evidence-based practices, innovative approaches, and a global perspective, it strives to position itself as a must-have reference for healthcare professionals and an indispensable guide for individuals seeking to take control of their skin health.

Ultimately, our goal is to contribute to the ongoing efforts to improve outcomes, minimize the burden of basal cell carcinoma, and enhance the quality of life for those affected by this condition. Join us on this journey as we unveil the complexities and conquer the challenge of basal cell carcinoma, one chapter at a time.

CHAPTER 1

Understanding Basal Cell Carcinoma

Basal cell carcinoma (BCC) is the most common form of skin cancer, affecting millions of individuals worldwide. As the name suggests, this malignancy originates from the basal cells, the lowest layer of the epidermis, the outermost part of the skin. Understanding the fundamental aspects of basal cell carcinoma, including its definition, classification, epidemiology, and underlying pathophysiology, is crucial for healthcare professionals and patients alike in the pursuit of effective prevention, early detection, and comprehensive management.

Defining Basal Cell Carcinoma

Basal cell carcinoma is a type of non-melanoma skin cancer that arises from the basal cells, which are responsible for continuously replenishing the skin's outermost layer. These basal cells are located in the deepest portion of the epidermis, known as the stratum basale. Under normal circumstances, the basal cells undergo controlled proliferation and differentiation to maintain the skin's structural integrity and protective function.

However, in the case of basal cell carcinoma, genetic alterations or environmental factors disrupt this delicate balance, leading to the uncontrolled proliferation of basal cells. As these abnormal cells multiply, they form a localized tumor or lesion, which can subsequently invade the surrounding tissues, including the dermis and even the underlying structures, such as muscle and bone.

Classifying Basal Cell Carcinoma

Basal cell carcinoma is not a single, homogeneous entity; rather, it encompasses a diverse spectrum of subtypes, each with its own distinct clinical characteristics and management considerations. Understanding the various BCC subtypes is crucial for accurate diagnosis, appropriate treatment selection, and optimizing patient outcomes.

The most commonly recognized subtypes of basal cell carcinoma include:

1. Nodular BCC: This is the most prevalent form, accounting for approximately 60-80% of all BCC cases. Nodular BCC typically presents as a well-defined, translucent or pearly, dome-shaped nodule with telangiectasias (visible blood vessels) on the surface.

2. Infiltrative BCC: Also known as morpheaform BCC, this subtype is characterized by an aggressive, infiltrative growth pattern that can extend deeply into the dermis and subcutaneous tissues. Infiltrative BCCs often appear as flat, scar-like lesions with indistinct borders, making them more challenging to detect and treat.

3. Superficial BCC: This subtype manifests as a flat, erythematous (reddish) plaque with a distinct border. Superficial BCCs tend to have a more indolent growth pattern and are often located on the trunk or extremities.

4. Micronodular BCC: This variant is characterized by the presence of multiple, small, discrete nodules that can coalesce to form a larger lesion. Micronodular BCCs have a higher risk of recurrence due to their infiltrative growth pattern.

5. Pigmented BCC: Some basal cell carcinomas can exhibit varying degrees of pigmentation, ranging from light tan to dark brown or black. This subtype may resemble melanoma, underscoring the importance of accurate diagnostic evaluation.

6. Basosquamous (Metatypical) BCC: This rare variant displays features of both basal cell carcinoma and squamous cell carcinoma, the second most common form of skin cancer. Basosquamous BCCs are considered more aggressive and have a higher risk of local invasion and metastasis.

It is important to note that these subtypes are not mutually exclusive, and a single BCC lesion may exhibit a combination of these characteristics. The recognition and accurate classification of BCC subtypes guide healthcare providers in selecting the most appropriate treatment strategies and tailoring management approaches to individual patient needs.

Epidemiology and Risk Factors

Basal cell carcinoma is the most common form of skin cancer, accounting for approximately 80% of all diagnosed skin cancers globally. The incidence of BCC has been steadily increasing over the past decades, driven by a complex interplay of environmental, genetic, and lifestyle factors.

Environmental Factors

Ultraviolet (UV) radiation exposure, particularly from natural sunlight and artificial sources like tanning beds, is the primary environmental risk factor for the development of basal cell carcinoma. UV radiation can induce DNA damage in the skin's basal cells, leading to genetic mutations and the subsequent uncontrolled proliferation of these cells.

Individuals with a history of chronic or intermittent sun exposure, particularly those with fair skin and a tendency to burn easily, are at a significantly higher risk of developing BCC. The anatomical location of BCC lesions often corresponds to areas of the body with the greatest sun exposure, such as the head, neck, and upper extremities.

Genetic Factors

Genetic predisposition also plays a crucial role in the development of basal cell carcinoma. Certain inherited genetic syndromes, such as Gorlin syndrome (also known as nevoid basal cell carcinoma syndrome or Gorlin-Goltz syndrome), are associated with an increased susceptibility to multiple, early-onset BCCs.

Gorlin syndrome is caused by mutations in the PTCH1 gene, which is a key regulator of the Hedgehog signaling pathway, a crucial developmental pathway implicated in the pathogenesis of BCC. Individuals with Gorlin syndrome often develop numerous BCCs, as well as other related conditions, such as odontogenic keratocysts and medulloblastoma.

In addition to Gorlin syndrome, certain genetic polymorphisms and mutations in other genes, such as TP53 and NOTCH1, have been linked to an increased risk of sporadic (non-syndromic) basal cell carcinoma. Understanding the genetic underpinnings of BCC is an area of active research, with the potential to inform personalized risk assessment and targeted preventive strategies.

Immunosuppression and Other Factors

Individuals with compromised immune systems, such as organ transplant recipients or those undergoing long-term immunosuppressive therapy, have a heightened risk of developing basal cell carcinoma and other non-melanoma skin cancers. The impairment of the immune system's ability to recognize and eliminate aberrant cells contributes to the increased susceptibility.

Furthermore, certain medications, such as arsenic-containing compounds and some chemotherapeutic agents, have been associated with an elevated risk of BCC development. Additionally, previous radiation therapy, chronic skin inflammation, and exposure to certain industrial chemicals have also been identified as potential risk factors for basal cell carcinoma.

Pathophysiology and Molecular Mechanisms

The development of basal cell carcinoma is a complex, multistep process involving the dysregulation of various signaling pathways and genetic alterations within the basal cells of the epidermis. Understanding the underlying pathophysiology of BCC is crucial for the development of novel diagnostic tools and targeted therapeutic strategies.

The Hedgehog Signaling Pathway

The Hedgehog signaling pathway is a fundamental developmental pathway that plays a pivotal role in the pathogenesis of basal cell carcinoma. This pathway is responsible for regulating cell growth, differentiation, and patterning during embryonic development and tissue homeostasis.

In healthy cells, the Hedgehog pathway is tightly regulated, with the PTCH1 gene acting as a negative regulator, inhibiting the activity of the SMO gene, a key component of the pathway. However, in basal cell carcinoma, mutations in the PTCH1 gene or other components of the Hedgehog signaling cascade can lead to the constitutive activation of this pathway, driving the uncontrolled proliferation of basal cells and the formation of a BCC lesion.

The importance of the Hedgehog pathway in BCC pathogenesis is under-scored by the fact that the majority of sporadic (non-syndromic) basal cell carcinomas harbor mutations in the PTCH1 gene or other Hedgehog-related genes, such as SMO and SUFU.

The p53 Tumor Suppressor Pathway

In addition to the Hedgehog signaling pathway, the p53 tumor suppressor pathway also plays a crucial role in the development of basal cell carcinoma. The p53 gene, known as the "guardian of the genome," is responsible for regulating cell cycle progression, DNA repair, and apoptosis (programmed cell death) in response to cellular stress or DNA damage.

In basal cell carcinoma, mutations or inactivation of the p53 gene can lead to the accumulation of genetically abnormal cells, impaired DNA repair mechanisms, and the evasion of apoptosis, all of which contribute to the uncontrolled proliferation of basal cells and the formation of a BCC lesion.

Furthermore, the interplay between the Hedgehog and p53 pathways has been the subject of extensive research in the field of BCC pathogenesis. Studies have suggested that the aberrant activation of the Hedgehog pathway can also lead to the inactivation of the p53 pathway, further exacerbating the malignant transformation of basal cells.

Other Signaling Pathways and Genetic Alterations

In addition to the Hedgehog and p53 pathways, other signaling cascades and genetic alterations have been implicated in the development of basal cell carcinoma. These include:

1. NOTCH signaling pathway: Dysregulation of the NOTCH pathway, which plays a role in cell fate determination and differentiation, has been associated with certain BCC subtypes.

2. RAS/MAPK pathway: Aberrant activation of the RAS/MAPK (mitogen-activated protein kinase) pathway, which is involved in cell proliferation and survival, has been observed in a subset of basal cell carcinomas.

3. Cell cycle regulators: Alterations in genes responsible for cell cycle control, such as CYCLIN D1 and CDKN2A, have been linked to the pathogenesis of BCC.

4. Epigenetic modifications: Changes in the epigenetic landscape, including DNA methylation and histone modifications, have been implicated in the dysregulation of gene expression patterns in basal cell carcinoma.

The complex interplay of these signaling pathways and genetic alterations underscores the heterogeneous nature of basal cell carcinoma and highlights the need for a personalized, multi-faceted approach to understanding and managing this disease.

Clinical Presentation and Progression

Basal cell carcinoma typically presents with a wide range of clinical manifestations, reflecting the diverse subtypes and the location of the lesions. Understanding the characteristic features of BCC is essential for healthcare providers to establish an accurate diagnosis and initiate appropriate treatment.

Nodular BCC, the most common subtype, often appears as a well-defined, translucent or pearly, dome-shaped nodule with telangiectasias (visible blood vessels) on the surface. These lesions may have a central depression or ulceration, known as a "rodent ulcer." Nodular BCCs are commonly found on sun-exposed areas, such as the face, head, and neck.

Infiltrative (morpheaform) BCC, on the other hand, presents as a flat, scar-like lesion with indistinct borders, making it challenging to detect and delineate the extent of the tumor. This subtype often infiltrates deeply into the dermis and surrounding tissues, increasing the risk of incomplete removal and recurrence.

Superficial BCC manifests as a flat, erythematous (reddish) plaque with a distinct border. These lesions tend to have a more indolent growth pattern and are typically located on the trunk or extremities.

Pigmented BCC can exhibit varying degrees of pigmentation, ranging from light tan to dark brown or black. This subtype may resemble melanoma, underscoring the importance of accurate diagnostic evaluation by a healthcare provider.

Basosquamous (metatypical) BCC, a rare variant, displays features of both basal cell carcinoma and squamous cell carcinoma, the second most common form of skin cancer. These lesions are considered more aggressive and have a higher risk of local invasion and metastasis.

In terms of progression, basal cell carcinoma is generally a slow-growing, locally invasive malignancy. However, if left untreated, BCC can progressively invade the surrounding tissues, including the dermis, subcutaneous fat, muscle, and even bone. In rare cases, BCC may also metastasize to distant sites, although this is an uncommon occurrence.

The rate of growth and the extent of local invasion can vary depending on the BCC subtype, the location of the lesion, and individual patient factors. Certain anatomical sites, such as the periocular region, nasal tip, and ears, are particularly prone to aggressive growth and local invasion due to the complex anatomy and limited surgical margins.

Accurate clinical recognition of the various BCC subtypes, combined with a thorough understanding of the potential for local invasion and progression, is essential for healthcare providers to develop effective treatment strategies and optimize patient outcomes.

Conclusion

Basal cell carcinoma is a complex and multifaceted skin malignancy that demands a comprehensive understanding of its definition, classification, epidemiology, and underlying pathophysiology. By delving into the intricacies of this common skin cancer, healthcare professionals and patients can better navigate the diagnostic landscape, implement tailored prevention strategies, and develop personalized management approaches.

The recognition of BCC subtypes, the identification of key risk factors, and the elucidation of the molecular mechanisms driving this disease are crucial steps in the pursuit of improved patient outcomes and quality of life. As the field of BCC research continues to evolve, the knowledge gained from this chapter will serve as a foundation for the subsequent exploration of diagnostic techniques, treatment modalities, and emerging innovations in the management of this pervasive skin cancer.

CHAPTER 2

Diagnosis and Clinical Presentation

Accurate and timely diagnosis of basal cell carcinoma (BCC) is the cornerstone of effective management and improved patient outcomes. Healthcare providers must be equipped with a comprehensive understanding of the various diagnostic modalities, from visual examination and dermatoscopy to biopsy and advanced imaging techniques. By mastering these diagnostic tools, clinicians can confidently differentiate BCC from other skin conditions, determine the specific subtype, and guide the most appropriate treatment approach.

In this chapter, we will delve into the multifaceted diagnostic landscape of basal cell carcinoma, empowering healthcare professionals and patients with the knowledge to navigate the complexities of this skin cancer.

Visual Examination and Dermatoscopy

The initial step in the diagnostic process for basal cell carcinoma often involves a thorough visual examination of the skin by a healthcare provider, typically a dermatologist or a trained primary care clinician. This comprehensive assessment allows for the identification of characteristic clinical features that can aid in the differential diagnosis.

During the visual examination, the clinician will carefully inspect the suspicious lesion, evaluating factors such as size, color, texture, and the presence of specific morphological features associated with basal cell carcinoma. Some of the hallmark characteristics of BCC include:

1. Pearly or waxy appearance: Basal cell carcinoma lesions often have a translucent, shiny, or "pearly" appearance, resembling a small, dome-shaped nodule.

2. Telangiectasias (visible blood vessels): The presence of fine, arborizing blood vessels on the surface of the lesion is a common finding in BCC.

3. Central ulceration or depression: Nodular BCCs frequently develop a central depression or ulceration, known as a "rodent ulcer."

4. Distinct borders: Many BCC lesions, particularly the nodular and superficial subtypes, have well-defined, distinct borders, in contrast to the more indistinct margins seen in infiltrative BCCs.

5. Pigmentation: While most BCCs appear pink or flesh-colored, a subset of these lesions can exhibit varying degrees of pigmentation, ranging from light tan to dark brown or black.

While visual examination provides invaluable information, the addition of dermatoscopy can significantly enhance the diagnostic accuracy for basal cell carcinoma. Dermatoscopy, also known as epiluminescence microscopy, involves the use of a handheld device equipped with a magnifying lens and polarized light source to examine the skin at a higher magnification.

The dermatoscopic features of basal cell carcinoma include:

1. Arborizing telangiectasias: The presence of fine, branching, tree-like blood vessels is a hallmark dermatoscopic sign of BCC.

2. Maple leaf-like structures: These well-defined, leaf-shaped, reddish-brown structures are often observed in nodular and superficial BCCs.

3. Blue-grey ovoid nests: Discrete, blue-grey, ovoid structures can be seen in some BCC lesions.

4. Spoke-wheel structures: Radially arranged, comma-shaped, whitish-pink structures resembling a wheel can be a distinctive dermatoscopic finding.

5. Ulceration and erosion: The presence of central ulceration or erosion is a common feature, particularly in nodular BCCs.

By incorporating dermatoscopic evaluation into the diagnostic process, healthcare providers can improve their ability to differentiate basal cell carcinoma from other skin conditions, such as benign nevi (moles), seborrheic keratosis, and squamous cell carcinoma. This enhanced diagnostic accuracy can lead to more targeted treatment planning and improved patient outcomes.

Biopsy and Histopathological Analysis

While visual examination and dermatoscopy can provide valuable clues regarding the nature of a suspicious skin lesion, a definitive diagnosis of basal cell carcinoma ultimately requires a biopsy and subsequent histopathological analysis.

The biopsy procedure involves the removal of a small sample of the lesion, either through a punch biopsy, shave biopsy, or excisional biopsy, depending on the size and location of the suspected BCC. This tissue sample is then processed and examined under a microscope by a pathologist, who will assess the histological features and confirm the diagnosis of basal cell carcinoma.

Histopathological evaluation of a BCC lesion typically reveals the following characteristic features:

1. Basaloid cells: Basal cell carcinoma is characterized by the proliferation of basaloid cells, which are small, round to oval cells with a high nuclear-to-cytoplasmic ratio and a uniform, dark-staining nucleus.

2. Palisading arrangement: The basaloid cells in BCC often exhibit a characteristic palisading pattern, where the cells are arranged in a parallel, orderly fashion at the periphery of the tumor nests.

3. Peripheral nuclear palisading: In addition to the overall palisading arrangement, the nuclei of the basal cells at the periphery of the tumor nests may also show a distinct palisading pattern.

4. Retraction artifact: The presence of a clear, empty space between the tumor cells and the surrounding stroma, known as a retraction artifact, is a common histological feature of basal cell carcinoma.

5. Subtype-specific features: Depending on the specific BCC subtype, the pathologist may observe additional histological characteristics, such as the infiltrative growth pattern of morpheaform BCC or the nesting arrangement of micronodular BCC.

The histopathological analysis not only confirms the diagnosis of basal cell carcinoma but also provides critical information about the specific subtype, which has important implications for the choice of treatment and the anticipated clinical course.

In some cases, the initial biopsy may not be sufficient to definitively determine the BCC subtype, particularly when dealing with a small or superficial lesion. In such instances, a more comprehensive excisional biopsy or Mohs micrographic surgery may be required to obtain a larger tissue sample and accurately characterize the tumor.

Imaging Techniques

While visual examination, dermatoscopy, and biopsy are the mainstays of basal cell carcinoma diagnosis, advances in imaging techniques have expanded the diagnostic toolbox and provided healthcare providers with additional valuable information.

High-Frequency Ultrasound (HFUS)

High-frequency ultrasound (HFUS) is a non-invasive imaging modality that can be used to assess the depth and extent of basal cell carcinoma lesions. By utilizing high-frequency sound waves, HFUS can generate detailed, real-time images of the skin and underlying structures, allowing clinicians to visualize the three-dimensional architecture of the BCC tumor.

HFUS can provide valuable information regarding the thickness and infiltrative growth pattern of the BCC, which is particularly useful in the evaluation of morpheaform or recurrent lesions. This imaging technique can also help guide the selection of the most appropriate treatment approach, such as determining the feasibility of surgical excision or the need for deeper tissue sampling.

Reflectance Confocal Microscopy (RCM)

Reflectance confocal microscopy (RCM) is an innovative imaging technology that allows for the in vivo, non-invasive visualization of the skin's cellular and sub-cellular structures at a high resolution, comparable to that of traditional histopathological examination.

By using a near-infrared laser beam focused on the skin, RCM can capture real-time, high-contrast images of the epidermis and superficial dermis, enabling the identification of specific cellular and architectural features associated with basal cell carcinoma. This technique can be particularly helpful in the diagnosis of pigmented BCCs, which may closely resemble other pigmented skin lesions on clinical and dermatoscopic examination.

The use of RCM in the diagnosis of BCC has demonstrated high sensitivity and specificity, potentially reducing the need for invasive biopsies in select cases. Additionally, RCM can assist in delineating the lateral and deep margins of the tumor, guiding the planning of surgical interventions or the selection of alternative treatment modalities.

Other Imaging Modalities

While HFUS and RCM are the most commonly employed advanced imaging techniques for basal cell carcinoma, other modalities, such as optical coherence tomography (OCT) and magnetic resonance imaging (MRI), have also been investigated for their potential diagnostic applications.

Optical coherence tomography utilizes near-infrared light to produce high-resolution, cross-sectional images of the skin, allowing for the visualization of the tumor's depth and architectural features. Similarly, MRI can provide valuable information about the extent of BCC infiltration, particularly in cases involving deep or challenging anatomical locations, such as the head and neck region.

The integration of these advanced imaging techniques into the diagnostic workflow can enhance the clinician's ability to accurately characterize basal cell carcinoma, optimize treatment planning, and improve patient outcomes. However, it is important to note that the availability and accessibility of these specialized imaging modalities may vary depending on the healthcare setting and the expertise of the care team.

Clinical Presentation and Differential Diagnosis

Basal cell carcinoma can manifest in a wide range of clinical presentations, reflecting the diverse subtypes and the location of the lesions. Understanding the characteristic features of BCC, as well as recognizing the potential for atypical or overlapping presentations, is crucial for healthcare providers to establish an accurate diagnosis and initiate appropriate management.

Nodular BCC, the most common subtype, typically appears as a well-defined, translucent or pearly, dome-shaped nodule with telangiectasias on the surface. These lesions may have a central depression or ulceration, known as a "rodent ulcer." Nodular BCCs are commonly found on sun-exposed areas, such as the face, head, and neck.

Infiltrative (morpheaform) BCC, on the other hand, presents as a flat, scar-like lesion with indistinct borders, making it challenging to detect and delineate the extent of the tumor. This subtype often infiltrates deeply into the dermis and surrounding tissues, increasing the risk of incomplete removal and recurrence.

Superficial BCC manifests as a flat, erythematous (reddish) plaque with a distinct border. These lesions tend to have a more indolent growth pattern and are typically located on the trunk or extremities.

Pigmented BCC can exhibit varying degrees of pigmentation, ranging from light tan to dark brown or black. This subtype may resemble melanoma, underscoring the importance of accurate diagnostic evaluation by a healthcare provider.

Basosquamous (metatypical) BCC, a rare variant, displays features of both basal cell carcinoma and squamous cell carcinoma, the second most common form of skin cancer. These lesions are considered more aggressive and have a higher risk of local invasion and metastasis.

It is important to note that the clinical presentation of basal cell carcinoma can sometimes overlap with other dermatological conditions, making the differential diagnosis a crucial step in the diagnostic process. Healthcare providers must be vigilant in distinguishing BCC from the following conditions:

1. Seborrheic keratosis: A benign, wart-like growth that can appear as a pigmented, raised lesion, sometimes resembling a nodular BCC.

2. Melanocytic nevus (mole): A benign pigmented lesion that can occasionally mimic the appearance of a pigmented BCC.

3. Actinic keratosis: A precancerous skin condition characterized by scaly, rough patches, which may be confused with superficial BCC.

4. Squamous cell carcinoma: The second most common type of skin cancer, which can share some clinical features with certain BCC subtypes.

5. Dermatofibroma: A benign, firm, button-like growth that can sometimes be mistaken for a nodular BCC.

6. Scar or granuloma: Certain inflammatory conditions or traumatic skin changes can present in a way that resembles an infiltrative BCC.

The accurate differentiation of basal cell carcinoma from these mimicking conditions requires a comprehensive clinical evaluation, including a thorough history, physical examination, and the judicious use of diagnostic tools such as dermatoscopy, biopsy, and advanced imaging techniques.

By mastering the recognition of BCC's diverse clinical presentations and the ability to distinguish it from other skin conditions, healthcare providers can ensure timely and accurate diagnosis, leading to the implementation of the most appropriate treatment strategies and improved patient outcomes.

Conclusion

The diagnosis of basal cell carcinoma is a multi-faceted process that requires a comprehensive understanding of various diagnostic modalities, from visual examination and dermatoscopy to biopsy and advanced imaging techniques. By leveraging these diagnostic tools, healthcare providers can accurately identify BCC lesions, determine the specific subtype, and guide the most appropriate management approach.

The integration of cutting-edge imaging technologies, such as high-frequency ultrasound and reflectance confocal microscopy, has expanded the diagnostic arsenal and enhanced the clinician's ability to visualize the depth and extent of BCC tumors. This, in turn, facilitates more informed treatment planning and improved patient outcomes.

Recognizing the diverse clinical presentations of basal cell carcinoma and differentiating it from mimicking skin conditions are essential skills for healthcare providers. By mastering these diagnostic competencies, clinicians can ensure timely and accurate diagnoses, leading to the implementation of personalized treatment strategies and optimizing the overall management of this common skin malignancy.

The knowledge and insights gained from this chapter will serve as a foundation for the subsequent exploration of treatment options, prevention strategies, and the importance of patient-centered care in the comprehensive management of basal cell carcinoma.

CHAPTER 3

Early Detection and Prevention

The key to successful management of basal cell carcinoma (BCC) lies in early detection and prevention. By empowering individuals to recognize the early signs of this common skin cancer and encouraging healthcare providers to incorporate routine skin examinations into standard practice, we can significantly improve patient outcomes and minimize the burden of this disease.

In this chapter, we will explore the pivotal role of skin self-examination, the importance of the primary care provider's involvement, and the strategies for effective screening and risk stratification. By equipping both patients and healthcare professionals with the necessary knowledge and tools, we can promote early detection and implement targeted prevention measures, ultimately reducing the incidence and impact of basal cell carcinoma.

Skin Self-Examination: Empowering Patients

Skin self-examination is a crucial component of early detection and prevention for basal cell carcinoma. By encouraging patients to regularly inspect their skin and become familiar with the appearance of their moles and other lesions, we can empower them to play an active role in the detection of suspicious changes that may indicate the presence of BCC.

The Importance of Skin Self-Examination

Regular skin self-examination can significantly enhance the likelihood of early detection, as basal cell carcinoma often presents with characteristic visual and tactile features that can be recognized by the patient. Early detection is particularly important, as BCC lesions that are identified and treated in their initial stages are more likely to respond to treatment, minimizing the risk of local invasion, tissue destruction, and potential disfigurement.

Furthermore, skin self-examination can foster a heightened awareness and sense of ownership over one's skin health, encouraging patients to seek timely medical attention for any suspicious changes. This proactive approach can lead to earlier diagnosis, improved treatment outcomes, and a better overall quality of life.

Techniques for Effective Skin Self-Examination

To perform an effective skin self-examination, patients should follow these key steps:

1. Examine the entire body: Patients should inspect all areas of the skin, including hard-to-see regions like the scalp, back, and behind the ears, using a full-length mirror or enlisting the help of a partner or family member.

2. Look for characteristic features: Patients should be educated on the visual and tactile characteristics of basal cell carcinoma, such as a pearly, translucent, or waxy nodule, the presence of telangiectasias (visible blood vessels), and any changes in the size, shape, or color of a lesion.

3. Palpate the skin: In addition to visual inspection, patients should gently feel their skin for any changes in texture, such as a hard, firm, or raised lesion that may indicate the presence of a BCC.

4. Document and monitor changes: Patients should keep a record of their skin self-examinations, noting the location, size, and appearance of any suspicious lesions. This will help them monitor for any changes over time and facilitate discussions with their healthcare provider.

5. Seek medical attention: If patients notice any new, changing, or concerning lesions during their skin self-examinations, they should promptly schedule an appointment with a healthcare provider, such as a dermatologist or a primary care clinician trained in skin cancer detection.

Empowering Patients through Education and Resources

Educating patients on the importance of skin self-examination and providing them with the necessary tools and resources is crucial for the success of this early detection strategy. Healthcare providers can play a pivotal role in this process by:

1. Incorporating skin self-examination education into routine clinical visits: During regular checkups or consultations, healthcare providers should take the time to demonstrate proper skin self-examination techniques and emphasize the importance of this practice.

2. Distributing educational materials: Clinicians can provide patients with informational brochures, posters, or digital resources that clearly outline the steps for effective skin self-examination and highlight the characteristic features of basal cell carcinoma.

3. Encouraging the use of self-examination aids: Patients may benefit from the use of devices such as handheld mirrors or phone applications that can facilitate a more thorough and systematic skin inspection.

4. Fostering a culture of skin health awareness: Healthcare providers can promote skin cancer awareness campaigns, support patient-oriented

educational initiatives, and collaborate with community organizations to amplify the message of early detection and prevention.

By empowering patients through education and equipping them with the necessary skills and resources, healthcare providers can empower individuals to take an active role in the early detection of basal cell carcinoma, ultimately improving patient outcomes and reducing the burden of this skin cancer.

The Role of the Primary Care Provider

Primary care providers, such as family medicine physicians, internal medicine specialists, and nurse practitioners, play a vital role in the early detection and prevention of basal cell carcinoma. As the first point of contact for many patients, these healthcare professionals have the opportunity to implement comprehensive skin cancer screening and educational strategies within their practices.

Incorporating Routine Skin Examinations

One of the key responsibilities of primary care providers in the context of basal cell carcinoma is the incorporation of routine skin examinations as part of standard patient care. This proactive approach can lead to the early identification of suspicious lesions, facilitating prompt referral to a dermatologist for further evaluation and management.

During a comprehensive skin examination, the primary care provider should:

1. Visually inspect the entire body surface for any suspicious lesions, paying particular attention to sun-exposed areas.
2. Palpate the skin to detect any hard, firm, or elevated growths that may indicate the presence of a BCC.
3. Educate the patient on the characteristic features of basal cell carcinoma

and the importance of skin self-examination.

4. Document the findings of the skin examination in the patient's medical record, including the location, size, and appearance of any suspicious lesions.

5. Provide appropriate guidance and timely referral to a dermatologist for further assessment and management, if necessary.

By incorporating these routine skin examinations into standard clinical practice, primary care providers can significantly enhance the early detection of basal cell carcinoma, leading to improved patient outcomes and reduced morbidity associated with this skin cancer.

Educating Patients on Prevention Strategies

In addition to performing skin examinations, primary care providers play a crucial role in educating patients on effective prevention strategies for basal cell carcinoma. This education should focus on:

1. Sun protection measures: Advising patients on the importance of sun avoidance, the use of broad-spectrum sunscreen, and the adoption of protective clothing and hats can help reduce the risk of developing BCC.

2. Skin self-examination: Promoting the practice of regular skin self-examinations and providing guidance on the techniques and characteristic features to look for can empower patients to be active participants in their skin health.

3. Risk factor awareness: Educating patients on the various risk factors for basal cell carcinoma, such as fair skin, a history of significant sun exposure, and certain genetic syndromes, can help them make informed decisions about their preventive strategies.

4. Encouraging regular skin cancer screenings: Primary care providers should emphasize the importance of routine skin cancer screenings, particularly for high-risk individuals, and facilitate timely referrals to dermatologists as needed.

By taking a proactive approach to skin cancer prevention and education, primary care providers can significantly contribute to the early detection and management of basal cell carcinoma, ultimately improving patient outcomes and reducing the overall burden of this disease.

Screening and Risk Stratification

Effective screening and risk stratification strategies are essential components of a comprehensive approach to the early detection and prevention of basal cell carcinoma. By identifying individuals at a heightened risk of developing BCC, healthcare providers can implement targeted surveillance and prevention measures, optimizing the utilization of limited resources and enhancing patient outcomes.

Risk Factors and Risk Stratification

Several factors have been identified as contributing to an increased risk of developing basal cell carcinoma. These risk factors include:

1. Skin type and sun exposure: Individuals with fair skin, a tendency to burn easily, and a history of significant, chronic, or intermittent sun exposure are at a higher risk of BCC.

2. Genetic predisposition: Certain inherited genetic syndromes, such as Gorlin syndrome, are associated with an elevated susceptibility to multiple, early-onset basal cell carcinomas.

3. Immunosuppression: Individuals with compromised immune systems,

such as organ transplant recipients or those undergoing long-term immuno-suppressive therapy, have a heightened risk of developing BCC and other non-melanoma skin cancers.

4. Prior history of skin cancer: Patients with a personal history of basal cell carcinoma or other types of skin cancer have an increased risk of developing additional lesions.

5. Certain medications and radiation exposure: Exposure to arsenic-containing compounds, certain chemotherapeutic agents, and previous radiation therapy can also contribute to an elevated BCC risk.

By considering these risk factors, healthcare providers can stratify patients into different risk categories, ranging from low-risk to high-risk. This risk stratification process allows for the implementation of tailored screening and prevention strategies, ensuring that high-risk individuals receive more frequent skin examinations, personalized education, and close follow-up.

Screening Strategies for Basal Cell Carcinoma

Screening for basal cell carcinoma can be performed through various approaches, depending on the patient's risk profile and the healthcare setting.

1. Opportunistic screening: During routine clinical visits, healthcare providers can incorporate a thorough skin examination as part of the standard preventive care protocol, regardless of the presenting complaint. This "opportunistic" screening can lead to the early detection of BCC lesions in asymptomatic patients.

2. Targeted screening: For individuals identified as being at a higher risk of developing basal cell carcinoma, healthcare providers can establish a more structured screening program, with regular, scheduled skin examinations and skin cancer checks.

3. Community-based initiatives: Outreach programs, such as skin cancer screening events in community centers, workplaces, or schools, can help expand access to BCC screening and raise awareness among the general population.

4. Telehealth and digital screening: The integration of telemedicine and digital imaging technologies, such as smartphone-based applications, can facilitate remote skin cancer screening and enhance the reach of BCC detection efforts, especially in areas with limited access to in-person dermatological care.

Regardless of the specific screening approach, the key to success lies in the collaboration between healthcare providers, patients, and the broader community. By fostering a culture of skin health awareness and empowering individuals to actively participate in their own care, we can significantly improve the early detection and prevention of basal cell carcinoma.

Addressing Health Disparities in BCC Screening

It is important to note that access to BCC screening and preventive services may be disproportionately limited for certain populations, particularly those from underserved or socioeconomically disadvantaged communities. Healthcare providers and policymakers must work to address these disparities and ensure equitable access to skin cancer detection and prevention initiatives.

Strategies to address health disparities in BCC screening may include:

1. Expanding telehealth and mobile screening programs: Leveraging digital technologies and bringing screening services directly to underserved communities can help bridge the access gap.

2. Engaging community-based organizations: Collaborating with local community groups, places of worship, and grassroots organizations can

facilitate the reach of screening efforts and foster trust within the targeted populations.

3. Providing language-appropriate and culturally relevant education: Tailoring educational materials and outreach campaigns to the specific needs and cultural preferences of diverse communities can improve engagement and acceptance of BCC screening.

4. Advocating for policy changes and increased funding: Advocating for policies and securing funding to support comprehensive skin cancer screening initiatives, particularly in underserved areas, can contribute to more equitable access to these services.

By addressing health disparities and ensuring that all individuals have access to effective BCC screening and prevention strategies, we can work towards reducing the burden of this common skin cancer and improving overall health outcomes for the entire population.

Conclusion

Early detection and prevention are the cornerstones of effective management for basal cell carcinoma. By empowering patients to become active participants in their skin health through skin self-examination, and by equipping primary care providers with the necessary tools and resources to incorporate routine skin cancer screening into their practices, we can significantly enhance the early identification of BCC lesions.

The implementation of targeted screening and risk stratification strategies, tailored to the individual's risk profile, further strengthens our efforts in the fight against basal cell carcinoma. By identifying high-risk individuals and providing them with personalized prevention and surveillance measures, we can optimize the utilization of healthcare resources and improve patient outcomes.

Lastly, addressing health disparities in BCC screening and prevention is crucial to ensure equitable access to these services, ultimately promoting better overall skin health and reducing the burden of this common skin malignancy across all communities.

As we move forward, the knowledge and strategies discussed in this chapter will serve as a foundation for the subsequent exploration of comprehensive treatment approaches, the importance of patient-centered care, and the ongoing research and innovations that are transforming the management of basal cell carcinoma.

CHAPTER 4

Surgical Treatment Options

Surgical intervention remains the mainstay of treatment for the majority of basal cell carcinoma (BCC) cases. The primary goal of surgical management is to achieve complete removal of the tumor while minimizing the risk of recurrence and optimizing cosmetic and functional outcomes for the patient. In this chapter, we will explore the various surgical techniques available for the treatment of basal cell carcinoma, their indications, and the key considerations that guide the selection of the most appropriate approach.

Excision and Mohs Micrographic Surgery

Surgical excision and Mohs micrographic surgery are the two most commonly employed surgical techniques for the treatment of basal cell carcinoma.

Surgical Excision

Surgical excision involves the removal of the entire BCC lesion, along with a margin of healthy surrounding tissue, to ensure complete elimination of the tumor. This approach is often the preferred treatment for smaller, well-defined, and less aggressive BCC subtypes, such as nodular and superficial BCCs.

The key steps in the surgical excision of a BCC lesion include:

1. Preoperative assessment: The healthcare provider (typically a dermatologist or a Mohs surgeon) will carefully examine the lesion, assess its size, location, and subtype, and determine the appropriate surgical margins.

2. Local anesthesia: The area surrounding the BCC lesion is numbed with a local anesthetic to ensure patient comfort during the procedure.

3. Surgical excision: The healthcare provider uses a scalpel to remove the entire BCC lesion, including a margin of healthy skin around the tumor, typically ranging from 3-5 millimeters in width.

4. Wound closure: The resulting surgical defect is then closed using sutures, skin grafts, or other reconstructive techniques, depending on the size and location of the excision.

5. Histopathological examination: The excised tissue is sent to a pathologist for microscopic analysis to confirm complete removal of the BCC.

The success of surgical excision is largely dependent on the accurate identification and removal of the entire tumor, including any subclinical extensions. Incomplete excision can lead to a higher risk of recurrence, necessitating additional treatment or a more extensive surgical approach.

Mohs Micrographic Surgery

Mohs micrographic surgery, also known as Mohs surgery, is a specialized surgical technique that offers the highest cure rates for the treatment of basal cell carcinoma. This procedure is particularly useful for high-risk or difficult-to-treat BCC lesions, such as those with a history of recurrence, located in cosmetically sensitive areas, or exhibiting an infiltrative growth pattern.

The key features of Mohs micrographic surgery include:

1. Tumor mapping and staged excision: The healthcare provider (a Mohs surgeon) first removes the visible portion of the BCC lesion, then methodically maps and removes additional layers of tissue in a stepwise fashion, examining each layer under a microscope to ensure complete tumor removal.

2. Intraoperative histopathological analysis: The excised tissue samples are processed and examined by the Mohs surgeon in real-time, allowing for the immediate identification and removal of any remaining tumor cells.

3. Precision and conservation of healthy tissue: The meticulous, layer-by-layer approach of Mohs surgery aims to remove the entire tumor while minimizing the amount of healthy tissue excised, optimizing cosmetic and functional outcomes.

4. High cure rates: Mohs micrographic surgery has been shown to have the highest reported cure rates for the treatment of basal cell carcinoma, with recurrence rates typically ranging from 1% to 5% for primary BCC and 5% to 10% for recurrent BCC.

The primary advantages of Mohs surgery over standard surgical excision include the ability to precisely map and remove the entire tumor, the conservation of healthy tissue, and the higher cure rates, particularly for high-risk or aggressive BCC subtypes.

However, it is important to note that Mohs surgery is a specialized procedure that requires extensive training and expertise. Not all healthcare facilities may have access to Mohs surgeons, which can limit the availability of this technique in certain geographic locations or healthcare settings.

Curettage and Electrodessication

Curettage and electrodessication, also known as C&E, is a surgical technique that involves the mechanical and thermal destruction of the BCC lesion. This approach is often considered for the treatment of smaller, well-defined, and less aggressive basal cell carcinomas, particularly in patients who may not be suitable candidates for more extensive surgical procedures.

The key steps in the C&E procedure include:

1. Anesthesia: The area surrounding the BCC lesion is numbed with a local anesthetic.

2. Curettage: The healthcare provider uses a sharp, spoon-shaped instrument called a curette to scrape and remove the visible portion of the BCC tumor.

3. Electrodessication: Immediately following curettage, an electrified needle is used to apply a controlled amount of heat to the treatment area, effectively destroying any remaining tumor cells.

4. Repeat curettage and electrodessication: The process of curettage and electrodessication may be repeated multiple times to ensure complete removal of the BCC lesion.

5. Wound care: The treated area is allowed to heal through secondary intention, with the healthcare provider monitoring the wound for any signs of recurrence or complications.

The advantages of curettage and electrodessication include its relative simplicity, shorter procedure time, and the ability to treat multiple lesions in a single session. However, this technique is generally reserved for specific BCC subtypes (e.g., superficial, nodular) and smaller lesions, as it may be less effective for larger, deeper, or more aggressive tumors.

The recurrence rates for C&E can range from 5% to 10% for primary BCC and up to 15% for recurrent BCC, which is higher than the rates observed with surgical excision or Mohs micrographic surgery. As a result, close follow-up and monitoring are essential for patients treated with this approach.

Cryotherapy and Laser Therapy

In addition to the more conventional surgical techniques, healthcare providers may also consider alternative methods, such as cryotherapy and laser therapy, for the management of select basal cell carcinoma cases.

Cryotherapy

Cryotherapy, or cryosurgery, involves the destruction of the BCC lesion through the application of extreme cold, typically using liquid nitrogen. This approach is often considered for the treatment of smaller, well-defined, and superficial BCC subtypes.

The key steps in cryotherapy for BCC include:

1. Anesthesia: The area surrounding the BCC lesion is numbed with a local anesthetic.
2. Cryogen application: Liquid nitrogen is applied directly to the BCC lesion using a specialized probe or spray device, causing the tumor cells to freeze and undergo cryonecrosis.
3. Freeze-thaw cycles: Depending on the size and depth of the BCC, the healthcare provider may repeat the freeze-thaw cycle multiple times to ensure complete destruction of the tumor.
4. Wound care: The treated area is allowed to heal, with the healthcare provider monitoring for any signs of recurrence or complications.

Cryotherapy can be a useful option for patients who may not be suitable candidates for more invasive surgical procedures, or for the treatment of smaller, low-risk BCC lesions. However, it is generally less effective for larger, deeper, or more aggressive BCC subtypes, and the recurrence rates can be higher compared to surgical excision or Mohs surgery.

Laser Therapy

Laser therapy, specifically the use of ablative lasers, has also been explored as a treatment option for select basal cell carcinoma cases. This approach involves the use of high-energy light beams to vaporize and destroy the BCC tumor.

The key steps in laser therapy for BCC include:

1. Anesthesia: The area surrounding the BCC lesion is numbed with a local anesthetic.
2. Laser application: The healthcare provider uses a specialized laser device to precisely target and ablate the BCC tumor, layer by layer.
3. Wound care: The treated area is allowed to heal, with the healthcare provider monitoring for any signs of recurrence or complications.

Laser therapy can be particularly useful for the treatment of superficial or small, well-defined BCC lesions, especially in cosmetically sensitive areas where scarring or disfigurement is a concern. However, like cryotherapy, laser therapy may be less effective for larger, deeper, or more aggressive BCC subtypes, and the recurrence rates can be higher than those observed with surgical excision or Mohs surgery.

Selecting the Appropriate Surgical Approach

The selection of the most appropriate surgical technique for the treatment of basal cell carcinoma depends on a variety of factors, including the size, location, and subtype of the BCC lesion, as well as the patient's individual characteristics and preferences.

Factors Influencing Surgical Treatment Selection

1. Tumor characteristics:
   - Size: Larger BCC lesions may require more extensive surgical approaches, such as Mohs micrographic surgery, to ensure complete tumor removal.
   - Location: BCC lesions in cosmetically sensitive areas or areas with limited surgical margins (e.g., periocular region, nasal tip) may benefit from Mohs surgery or other techniques that prioritize tissue preservation.
   - Subtype: Aggressive BCC subtypes, such as infiltrative or morpheaform, may require more specialized surgical techniques to address the potential for deep tissue invasion.

2. Patient factors:
   - Age and overall health status: Older patients or those with significant comorbidities may be better suited for less invasive surgical options or alternative treatment modalities.
   - Tumor recurrence history: Patients with a history of recurrent BCC may benefit from Mohs surgery or other more extensive surgical approaches to minimize the risk of further recurrence.
   - Cosmetic and functional considerations: Patients who place a high priority on optimizing cosmetic outcomes or preserving function (e.g., in the head and neck region) may be better candidates for Mohs surgery or reconstructive techniques.

3. Healthcare provider expertise and setting:
   - Availability of Mohs surgeons: The presence of a Mohs surgeon in the healthcare facility can influence the selection of this specialized surgical technique.
   - Surgical experience and training: The healthcare provider's level of

expertise and training in various surgical techniques may guide the choice of the most appropriate approach.

- Healthcare facility resources: The availability of specialized equipment, staffing, and support services can also impact the selection of the surgical approach.

Surgical Treatment Algorithms and Guidelines

To assist healthcare providers in the decision-making process, various professional organizations and clinical guidelines have developed algorithms and recommendations for the surgical management of basal cell carcinoma.

These guidelines generally consider the following factors when recommending the most appropriate surgical approach:

1. Tumor characteristics:
   - Size: Lesions larger than 2 cm in diameter may be better suited for Mohs surgery or other more extensive surgical techniques.
   - Location: Lesions in high-risk anatomical locations, such as the head and neck region, may warrant Mohs surgery or careful consideration of surgical margins.
   - Subtype: Aggressive BCC subtypes, such as infiltrative or morpheaform, are often recommended for Mohs surgery or excision with wider surgical margins.

2. Patient factors:
   - History of recurrence: Patients with a history of recurrent BCC are typically recommended for Mohs surgery or more extensive surgical approaches.
   - Comorbidities and life expectancy: Older patients or those with significant health conditions may be better candidates for less invasive surgical options or alternative treatments.

3. Healthcare provider expertise and setting:

- Availability of Mohs surgeons: If a Mohs surgeon is available, this specialized technique is often recommended for high-risk or difficult-to-treat BCC lesions.

- Surgical experience and training: The healthcare provider's level of expertise in various surgical techniques should be considered when selecting the most appropriate approach.

By considering these factors and following evidence-based guidelines, healthcare providers can make informed decisions and select the surgical treatment option that is most likely to achieve complete tumor removal, minimize the risk of recurrence, and optimize cosmetic and functional outcomes for the patient.

Conclusion

Surgical intervention remains the mainstay of treatment for the majority of basal cell carcinoma cases. The selection of the appropriate surgical approach, be it excision, Mohs micrographic surgery, curettage and electrodessication, or alternative techniques like cryotherapy and laser therapy, is crucial in delivering effective and personalized care to patients with BCC.

Healthcare providers must carefully consider the characteristics of the BCC lesion, the patient's individual factors, and the available resources and expertise within their healthcare setting to determine the most suitable surgical approach. By following evidence-based guidelines and algorithms, clinicians can optimize the balance between oncological control, cosmetic outcomes, and functional preservation.

As advancements continue to shape the surgical management of basal cell carcinoma, healthcare providers must remain vigilant in staying up-to-date with the latest techniques, guidelines, and best practices. This commitment to excellence in surgical care will ultimately lead to improved patient outcomes and a reduction in the burden of this common skin cancer.

The knowledge and insights gained from this chapter will serve as a foundation for the subsequent exploration of non-surgical treatment options, the management of advanced and metastatic BCC, and the importance of patient-centered care in the comprehensive approach to basal cell carcinoma.

CHAPTER 5

Non-Surgical Treatments

While surgical intervention remains the mainstay of basal cell carcinoma (BCC) management, a growing array of non-surgical treatment options have emerged as valuable alternatives, particularly for select patient populations and specific clinical scenarios. These non-surgical approaches offer the potential for effective tumor control, improved cosmetic outcomes, and enhanced patient satisfaction.

In this chapter, we will explore the various non-surgical treatment modalities available for the management of basal cell carcinoma, including topical medications, photodynamic therapy, and radiation therapy. We will delve into the mechanisms of action, indications, and the relative advantages and limitations of each approach, empowering healthcare providers to make informed decisions and personalize the care for their patients with BCC.

Topical Medications

Topical medications have become an increasingly important component in the non-surgical management of basal cell carcinoma, particularly for select subtypes and patient populations.

Imiquimod

Imiquimod is a topical immune-response modifier that has been approved for the treatment of superficial basal cell carcinoma. This medication works by stimulating the body's immune system, triggering the release of cytokines and other inflammatory mediators that can directly target and destroy the BCC tumor cells.

The key features of imiquimod therapy for BCC include:

1. Application and dosing: Imiquimod is typically applied to the affected area once daily, 2-3 times per week, for a specified duration (typically 6-12 weeks) as directed by the healthcare provider.

2. Mechanism of action: Imiquimod activates Toll-like receptors on immune cells, leading to the release of cytokines, such as interferon-alpha and tumor necrosis factor-alpha, which can induce apoptosis (programmed cell death) in the BCC tumor cells.

3. Efficacy: Studies have reported complete clearance rates for superficial BCC ranging from 70% to 90% with imiquimod therapy, making it a viable alternative to surgical approaches for select patients.

4. Advantages: Imiquimod offers a non-invasive, cosmetically attractive treatment option, particularly for patients with multiple or recurrent superficial BCCs or those who wish to avoid surgery.

5. Limitations: Imiquimod is primarily indicated for the treatment of superficial BCC and may be less effective for other BCC subtypes, such as nodular or infiltrative lesions. Additionally, the prolonged application period and potential for local skin reactions (e.g., erythema, crusting, erosion) can be a challenge for some patients.

5-Fluorouracil (5-FU)

5-Fluorouracil (5-FU) is another topical medication that has been utilized in the management of basal cell carcinoma. This antimetabolite agent interferes with the synthesis of DNA and RNA, leading to the selective destruction of rapidly dividing tumor cells.

The key features of 5-FU therapy for BCC include:

1. Application and dosing: 5-FU is typically applied to the affected area twice daily for a duration of 2-4 weeks, as directed by the healthcare provider.

2. Mechanism of action: 5-FU is preferentially absorbed and metabolized by rapidly dividing cells, such as BCC tumor cells, leading to the inhibition of DNA and RNA synthesis and ultimately inducing cell death.

3. Efficacy: Studies have reported complete clearance rates for superficial and nodular BCC ranging from 70% to 80% with 5-FU therapy.

4. Advantages: Like imiquimod, 5-FU offers a non-invasive treatment option, particularly for patients with multiple or recurrent BCC lesions or those who wish to avoid surgery.

5. Limitations: 5-FU therapy may be less effective for more aggressive BCC subtypes, such as infiltrative or morpheaform lesions. The treatment course can also be associated with significant local skin reactions, including erythema, inflammation, and pain, which can be a challenge for some patients.

Combination Therapy with Topical Medications

In some cases, healthcare providers may consider combining topical medications, such as imiquimod and 5-FU, to enhance the treatment efficacy for basal cell carcinoma. The rationale behind this approach is to target the tumor cells through different mechanisms of action, potentially improving the overall clearance rates and patient outcomes.

Studies have suggested that combination therapy with imiquimod and 5-FU can be more effective than either agent alone, particularly for the treatment of high-risk or recurrent BCC lesions. However, the increased intensity of the treatment course and the potential for more severe local skin reactions must be carefully weighed against the potential benefits.

Patient selection and close monitoring are crucial when considering combination topical therapy, as the enhanced treatment effects may also lead to a higher incidence of adverse events and reduced tolerability for some individuals.

Photodynamic Therapy (PDT)

Photodynamic therapy (PDT) is a non-invasive treatment approach that utilizes the combination of a photosensitizing agent and targeted exposure to a specific wavelength of light to selectively destroy basal cell carcinoma tumor cells.

The key steps in the photodynamic therapy process for BCC include:

1. Photosensitizer application: A topical photosensitizing agent, such as aminolevulinic acid (ALA) or methyl aminolevulinate (MAL), is applied to the BCC lesion, where it is preferentially absorbed by the rapidly dividing tumor cells.

2. Incubation period: After the application of the photosensitizer, a specified incubation period (typically 1-3 hours) allows for the agent to be selectively accumulated in the BCC tumor cells.

3. Light exposure: Following the incubation period, the affected area is exposed to a specific wavelength of light, typically using a specialized LED or laser device. This light activation of the photosensitizer triggers the generation of reactive oxygen species, which can induce apoptosis and

necrosis of the BCC tumor cells.

4. Wound healing: The treated area is allowed to heal, with the healthcare provider monitoring for any signs of tumor recurrence or complications.

The advantages of photodynamic therapy for basal cell carcinoma include its non-invasive nature, the potential for improved cosmetic outcomes compared to surgical approaches, and the ability to treat multiple lesions simultaneously. PDT has been shown to be particularly effective for the management of superficial and nodular BCC subtypes, with reported complete clearance rates ranging from 70% to 90%.

However, PDT is not without its limitations. The treatment can be associated with significant pain and discomfort during the light exposure phase, and certain patient factors, such as the location and size of the BCC lesion, may influence the suitability and efficacy of this approach. Additionally, the availability and accessibility of specialized PDT equipment and trained healthcare providers can vary, limiting the widespread adoption of this treatment modality in some healthcare settings.

Radiation Therapy

Radiation therapy, either in the form of external beam radiation or brachytherapy (internal radiation), can be a valuable non-surgical treatment option for select cases of basal cell carcinoma.

External Beam Radiation Therapy

External beam radiation therapy involves the use of a linear accelerator to deliver targeted, high-energy radiation to the BCC lesion, with the goal of destroying the tumor cells while minimizing the impact on surrounding healthy tissues.

The key features of external beam radiation therapy for BCC include:

1. Treatment planning: The healthcare provider (typically a radiation oncologist) will carefully plan the radiation treatment, taking into account the size, location, and depth of the BCC lesion, as well as the patient's individual factors and preferences.

2. Fractionation and delivery: The total radiation dose is typically delivered in multiple, smaller fractions over the course of several treatment sessions, often spanning 4-6 weeks.

3. Efficacy: Studies have reported complete clearance rates for BCC ranging from 80% to 95% with external beam radiation therapy, particularly for smaller, well-defined lesions.

4. Advantages: Radiation therapy can be a suitable alternative for patients who are not candidates for surgery or who wish to avoid the potential scarring associated with surgical interventions.

5. Limitations: Radiation therapy may have a higher risk of long-term adverse effects, such as skin atrophy, telangiectasia, and the potential for secondary malignancies in younger patients. The availability of specialized radiation oncology services can also be a limiting factor in some healthcare settings.

Brachytherapy

Brachytherapy, a form of internal radiation therapy, involves the direct application of a radioactive source to the BCC lesion, allowing for the targeted delivery of the radiation dose while minimizing the exposure to surrounding healthy tissues.

The key features of brachytherapy for BCC include:

1. Treatment planning: The healthcare provider (typically a radiation oncologist) will carefully plan the brachytherapy treatment, taking into account the size, location, and depth of the BCC lesion, as well as the patient's individual factors and preferences.

2. Radioactive source implantation: The radioactive source, such as a small, sealed radiation seed or a flexible applicator, is placed directly on or within the BCC lesion, either temporarily or permanently.

3. Efficacy: Studies have reported complete clearance rates for BCC ranging from 85% to 95% with brachytherapy, particularly for smaller, well-defined lesions.

4. Advantages: Brachytherapy can offer a more targeted and localized radiation approach, potentially reducing the risk of long-term adverse effects compared to external beam radiation therapy.

5. Limitations: Brachytherapy may be less suitable for larger or deeper BCC lesions, and the availability of specialized brachytherapy services can be a limiting factor in some healthcare settings.

Patient Selection and Considerations for Non-Surgical Treatments

The selection of the most appropriate non-surgical treatment modality for basal cell carcinoma is based on a careful evaluation of various patient and tumor-specific factors, as well as the expertise and resources available within the healthcare setting.

Patient Factors

1. Age and life expectancy: Older patients or those with significant comorbidities may be better suited for non-surgical treatments, particularly if the risks associated with surgery outweigh the potential benefits.

2. Tumor location and size: Lesions in cosmetically sensitive areas or larger BCCs may be more suitable for non-surgical approaches that prioritize tissue preservation and favorable cosmetic outcomes.

3. Patient preferences and tolerability: Some patients may prefer non-surgical options, especially if they are concerned about the potential for scarring, disfigurement, or the invasive nature of surgical interventions.

4. Prior treatment history: Patients with a history of recurrent BCC or those who have previously undergone surgical interventions may benefit from the consideration of non-surgical treatment modalities.

Tumor Characteristics

1. Subtype and growth pattern: Superficial and nodular BCC subtypes are generally more responsive to non-surgical treatments, such as topical medications and photodynamic therapy, compared to more aggressive, infiltrative subtypes.

2. Tumor size and depth: Larger or deeper BCC lesions may require more specialized non-surgical approaches, such as external beam radiation therapy or brachytherapy, to ensure adequate tumor control.

3. Anatomical location: Lesions in cosmetically sensitive areas or with limited surgical margins (e.g., periocular region, nasal tip) may be better suited for non-surgical treatments that can preserve tissue and minimize disfigurement.

Healthcare Setting and Provider Expertise

1. Availability of specialized equipment and services: The accessibility of specialized equipment and the presence of trained healthcare providers (e.g., Mohs surgeons, radiation oncologists) can significantly influence the selection of non-surgical treatment options.

2. Interdisciplinary collaboration: The integration of various healthcare specialists, such as dermatologists, radiation oncologists, and plastic surgeons, can facilitate a comprehensive, multidisciplinary approach to non-surgical BCC management.

By carefully considering these patient, tumor, and healthcare setting factors, healthcare providers can make informed decisions and select the non-surgical treatment modality that offers the best balance of therapeutic efficacy, cosmetic outcomes, and patient preferences for individuals with basal cell carcinoma.

Conclusion

The non-surgical treatment options available for basal cell carcinoma, including topical medications, photodynamic therapy, and radiation therapy, have emerged as valuable alternatives to traditional surgical interventions. These approaches offer the potential for effective tumor control, improved cosmetic outcomes, and enhanced patient satisfaction in select clinical scenarios.

Healthcare providers must carefully evaluate the patient's individual characteristics, the specific features of the BCC lesion, and the available resources and expertise within their healthcare setting to determine the most appropriate non-surgical treatment strategy. By thoughtfully integrating these non-surgical modalities into the comprehensive management of basal cell carcinoma, clinicians can provide personalized, patient-centered care and optimize outcomes for individuals affected by this common skin cancer.

As the field of non-surgical BCC management continues to evolve, healthcare providers must stay abreast of the latest advancements, guidelines, and best practices to ensure they can offer their patients the full spectrum of treatment options. The knowledge and insights gained from this chapter will serve as a foundation for the subsequent exploration of the management of advanced and metastatic BCC, as well as the importance of patient education and shared decision-making in the holistic care of individuals with this condition.

55

CHAPTER 6

Advanced and Metastatic Basal Cell Carcinoma

While the majority of basal cell carcinomas (BCCs) are considered to have a relatively favorable prognosis when diagnosed and treated early, a small subset of these tumors can exhibit an aggressive, advanced, or even metastatic behavior. These rare, high-risk BCC cases represent a significant challenge in the management of this common skin cancer, requiring a specialized and multidisciplinary approach to achieve optimal outcomes.

In this chapter, we will delve into the complexities of advanced and metastatic basal cell carcinoma, exploring the factors that contribute to these atypical presentations, the unique diagnostic and management considerations, and the emerging targeted therapies that are revolutionizing the care of these challenging cases.

Identifying Advanced and Metastatic Basal Cell Carcinoma

Advanced basal cell carcinoma is generally defined as a tumor that has either locally invaded deeply into the surrounding tissues, including the muscles, bones, or vital structures, or has metastasized to distant sites, such as the lymph nodes or internal organs. These high-risk BCC cases are relatively uncommon, representing only a small percentage of all diagnosed BCCs, but they can have a significant impact on patient prognosis and quality of life.

The key characteristics that distinguish advanced or metastatic basal cell carcinoma include:

1. Extensive local invasion: BCC lesions that have infiltrated deeply into the surrounding tissues, such as the muscles, bones, or nerves, beyond the typical depth of a standard BCC.

2. Recurrence after multiple prior treatments: Patients with a history of recurrent BCC, particularly after previous surgical or non-surgical interventions, may be at an increased risk of developing an advanced or aggressive form of the disease.

3. Large tumor size: Basal cell carcinomas that have grown to an exceptionally large size, often exceeding 5 cm in diameter, may be more likely to exhibit advanced characteristics.

4. Certain histological subtypes: Aggressive BCC subtypes, such as infiltrative, morpheaform, or basosquamous, have a higher propensity for deep tissue invasion and a more challenging clinical course.

5. Metastatic spread: In rare cases, basal cell carcinoma can metastasize to distant sites, such as the lymph nodes, lungs, or other organs, posing a significant threat to the patient's health and survival.

Recognizing these key features is crucial for healthcare providers to identify high-risk BCC cases and initiate prompt, specialized management strategies to optimize patient outcomes.

Diagnostic Considerations for Advanced BCC

The accurate diagnosis and comprehensive evaluation of advanced or metastatic basal cell carcinoma require a multifaceted approach, involving a combination of clinical assessment, advanced imaging techniques, and, in some cases, specialized biopsy or molecular testing.

Clinical Evaluation

A thorough clinical examination, including a detailed history and a comprehensive physical assessment, is the foundation of the diagnostic process for advanced BCC. Healthcare providers should carefully evaluate the size, location, and characteristics of the primary tumor, as well as any signs of local invasion or regional lymph node involvement.

Advanced Imaging Modalities

The use of advanced imaging techniques, such as high-frequency ultrasound (HFUS), computed tomography (CT), magnetic resonance imaging (MRI), and positron emission tomography (PET), can provide valuable information about the extent of the BCC tumor, the depth of invasion, and the potential for metastatic spread.

1. High-frequency ultrasound (HFUS): HFUS can be particularly useful in assessing the depth of tumor invasion and identifying any involvement of deeper structures, such as muscles or bones.

2. Computed tomography (CT) and magnetic resonance imaging (MRI): These modalities can provide detailed, cross-sectional imaging of the primary tumor and any potential extension into surrounding tissues or organs.

3. Positron emission tomography (PET): PET scans, often combined with CT (PET/CT), can be utilized to detect the presence of distant metastases, which may not be evident on clinical examination or other imaging studies.

The selection of the most appropriate imaging technique(s) will depend on the specific clinical scenario and the anatomical location of the advanced BCC lesion.

Biopsy and Molecular Testing

In some cases, a biopsy of the primary tumor or suspected metastatic site may be necessary to confirm the diagnosis and characterize the histological subtype of the advanced basal cell carcinoma. This information can guide the selection of the most appropriate treatment strategy.

Additionally, emerging molecular testing, such as genetic profiling or the analysis of specific biomarkers, may provide valuable insights into the underlying biology of the advanced BCC tumor. These molecular techniques can help identify potential therapeutic targets and inform the use of targeted therapies, particularly in the management of metastatic or recurrent disease.

Multidisciplinary Collaboration

The management of advanced or metastatic basal cell carcinoma often requires a multidisciplinary approach, involving healthcare providers from various specialties, including dermatologists, oncologists, radiation oncologists, plastic surgeons, and palliative care specialists. This collaborative effort ensures a comprehensive evaluation of the patient's condition and the development of a personalized treatment plan that addresses the unique challenges presented by the advanced BCC.

Treatment Strategies for Advanced and Metastatic BCC

The management of advanced and metastatic basal cell carcinoma can be complex and may involve a combination of surgical, non-surgical, and systemic treatment modalities. The primary goals of treatment are to achieve local control of the tumor, prevent or manage metastatic spread, and optimize the patient's quality of life.

Surgical Intervention

For select cases of advanced basal cell carcinoma, surgical excision may still be a viable treatment option, particularly if the tumor is localized and there is a reasonable expectation of complete removal with adequate surgical margins. However, the complexity of these cases often requires the expertise of a multidisciplinary surgical team, including Mohs surgeons, plastic surgeons, and reconstructive specialists.

In situations where the tumor has extensively invaded the surrounding tissues or vital structures, such as the skull base or orbital region, a more extensive surgical approach, including the removal of affected muscles, bones, or nerves, may be necessary. These complex procedures carry a higher risk of complications and may have significant functional and cosmetic implications for the patient, necessitating a careful evaluation of the risks and benefits.

Non-Surgical Modalities

When surgical intervention is not feasible or has been exhausted, healthcare providers may consider alternative non-surgical treatment options for advanced or metastatic basal cell carcinoma, such as:

1. Radiation therapy: External beam radiation therapy or brachytherapy can be used to target the primary tumor or metastatic lesions, with the goal of achieving local control and palliating symptoms.

2. Topical medications: In some cases, topical therapies, such as imiquimod or 5-fluorouracil, may be considered as an adjunct or alternative treatment for select advanced BCC lesions.

3. Photodynamic therapy (PDT): The use of photosensitizing agents and targeted light exposure can be a valuable non-invasive approach for the management of certain advanced BCC cases.

The selection of the most appropriate non-surgical modality will depend on the specific characteristics of the advanced BCC, the patient's overall health and preferences, and the expertise available within the healthcare setting.

Systemic Therapies: Hedgehog Pathway Inhibitors

The advent of targeted systemic therapies, specifically the class of medications known as Hedgehog pathway inhibitors, has revolutionized the management of advanced and metastatic basal cell carcinoma.

The Hedgehog signaling pathway plays a crucial role in the pathogenesis of the majority of basal cell carcinomas, as discussed in Chapter 1. Aberrant activation of this pathway, often due to mutations in key regulatory genes, such as PTCH1 and SMO, is a common driver of BCC tumor growth and proliferation.

Hedgehog pathway inhibitors, such as vismodegib and sonidegib, have been specifically developed to target and disrupt the Hedgehog signaling cascade, effectively inhibiting the growth and progression of BCC tumors.

The key features of Hedgehog pathway inhibitor therapy for advanced and metastatic basal cell carcinoma include:

1. Mechanism of action: These targeted agents bind to and inhibit the Smoothened (SMO) protein, a key component of the Hedgehog signaling pathway, thereby preventing the activation of this oncogenic cascade.

2. Efficacy: Studies have demonstrated that Hedgehog pathway inhibitors can achieve significant tumor regression and disease control in patients with advanced, inoperable, or metastatic basal cell carcinoma, with reported response rates ranging from 30% to 50%.

3. Dosing and administration: Hedgehog pathway inhibitors are typically administered orally, with the dosage and duration of treatment tailored to

the individual patient's response and tolerability.

4. Adverse effects: These targeted therapies can be associated with a range of adverse effects, including muscle spasms, alopecia, dysgeusia (taste disturbances), and fatigue, which must be closely monitored and managed by the healthcare team.

The availability of Hedgehog pathway inhibitors has significantly expanded the treatment options for patients with advanced or metastatic basal cell carcinoma, particularly in situations where traditional surgical or non-surgical approaches are no longer feasible or have been exhausted.

Combination Therapy Approaches

In some cases, healthcare providers may consider combining Hedgehog pathway inhibitors with other treatment modalities, such as radiation therapy or surgical intervention, to enhance the effectiveness of the management strategy for advanced or metastatic basal cell carcinoma.

The rationale for combination therapy is to leverage the complementary mechanisms of action and potentially achieve improved tumor control, while also mitigating the risk of treatment resistance or disease progression. However, the selection of the appropriate combination approach and the careful management of potential adverse effects require close collaboration within a multidisciplinary team.

Palliative and Supportive Care

For patients with advanced or metastatic basal cell carcinoma who are not candidates for curative-intent treatment or have exhausted all available treatment options, the focus of care shifts towards palliative and supportive measures to optimize the patient's quality of life.

This may include:

1. Symptom management: Providing relief for pain, bleeding, disfigurement, or other distressing symptoms associated with the advanced BCC tumor.
2. Wound care: Implementing specialized wound management protocols to address any ulceration, necrosis, or infection at the tumor site.
3. Psychosocial support: Offering counseling, support groups, and other resources to address the emotional and psychological impact of advanced disease.
4. Coordination of hospice or palliative care services: Referral to specialized palliative care teams to provide comprehensive, holistic support for the patient and their family.

By incorporating a palliative care approach, healthcare providers can ensure that patients with advanced or metastatic basal cell carcinoma receive compassionate, symptom-focused care and maintain the best possible quality of life during the later stages of their disease.

Monitoring and Follow-up

Regardless of the treatment approach, close monitoring and follow-up are crucial for patients with advanced or metastatic basal cell carcinoma. Regular clinical examinations, imaging studies, and laboratory tests are essential to:

1. Assess the response to treatment and detect any signs of disease progression or recurrence.
2. Identify and manage any treatment-related adverse effects or complications.
3. Provide timely adjustments to the treatment plan and coordinate

additional supportive care as needed.

The frequency and intensity of the monitoring and follow-up schedule will depend on the specific characteristics of the advanced BCC, the treatment modalities employed, and the overall health and clinical status of the patient.

Collaborative, Multidisciplinary Care

The management of advanced and metastatic basal cell carcinoma requires a collaborative, multidisciplinary approach, involving healthcare providers from various specialties, including dermatologists, oncologists, radiation oncologists, plastic surgeons, and palliative care specialists. This integrated care model ensures a comprehensive evaluation of the patient's condition, the development of a personalized treatment plan, and the coordination of the various components of care.

By fostering this interdisciplinary collaboration, healthcare providers can leverage their collective expertise, optimize the utilization of available resources, and provide the most comprehensive and personalized care for patients with advanced or metastatic basal cell carcinoma.

Conclusion

Advanced and metastatic basal cell carcinoma, while relatively uncommon, represent a significant challenge in the management of this common skin cancer. These high-risk cases require a specialized and multidisciplinary approach to achieve optimal outcomes, drawing on a combination of surgical, non-surgical, and systemic treatment modalities.

The accurate identification of advanced BCC, through a thorough clinical evaluation and the judicious use of advanced imaging and molecular testing, is the foundation for the development of an effective management strategy.

The selection of the appropriate treatment approach must take into account the specific characteristics of the tumor, the patient's overall health and preferences, and the available expertise and resources within the healthcare setting.

The advent of targeted Hedgehog pathway inhibitors has revolutionized the care of advanced and metastatic basal cell carcinoma, offering new hope and improved outcomes for patients with these challenging cases. However, the management of advanced BCC continues to evolve, and healthcare providers must remain vigilant in staying up-to-date with the latest advancements, evidence-based guidelines, and best practices to provide the most comprehensive and personalized care for their patients.

The knowledge and insights gained from this chapter will serve as a framework for the subsequent exploration of special considerations in BCC management, the importance of cosmetic and functional outcomes, and the emerging trends and future directions in the field of basal cell carcinoma care.

CHAPTER 7

Special Considerations

While basal cell carcinoma (BCC) is a common skin cancer with generally favorable outcomes when detected and treated early, there are specific clinical scenarios and patient populations that require additional considerations and tailored management approaches. In this chapter, we will explore some of these special circumstances, including the management of BCC in unique anatomical locations, the unique challenges presented by hereditary syndromes, and the considerations for immunosuppressed patients.

Basal Cell Carcinoma in Unique Anatomical Locations

Certain anatomical regions of the body pose unique challenges in the management of basal cell carcinoma, often due to the complex anatomy, limited surgical margins, or the potential for functional and cosmetic implications.

Periocular Region

Basal cell carcinomas located in the periocular region, including the eyelids, canthi, and orbital area, require specialized attention and a multidisciplinary approach. These lesions are particularly challenging due to the delicate nature of the surrounding structures, the potential for local tissue invasion, and the importance of preserving visual function and cosmetic outcomes.

Key management considerations for periocular BCCs include:

1. Thorough clinical evaluation: A comprehensive examination, including a slit-lamp examination, is essential to assess the extent of the tumor and its relationship to critical structures, such as the lacrimal system, eyelid margins, and the orbital contents.

2. Specialized diagnostic techniques: Advanced imaging modalities, such as high-frequency ultrasound (HFUS) and magnetic resonance imaging (MRI), can provide valuable information about the depth of tumor invasion and aid in surgical planning.

3. Multidisciplinary collaboration: The management of periocular BCCs often requires a collaborative effort between dermatologists, ophthalmologists, oculoplastic surgeons, and radiation oncologists to ensure the optimal balance between complete tumor removal and the preservation of function and cosmetic outcomes.

4. Specialized surgical techniques: Surgical approaches for periocular BCCs, such as Mohs micrographic surgery, may be modified to accommodate the unique anatomy and minimize the risk of complications, including visual impairment, ectropion, and lacrimal system dysfunction.

5. Alternative treatment modalities: In select cases, non-surgical options, such as radiation therapy or topical medications, may be considered when surgical intervention poses a high risk of significant functional or cosmetic impairment.

Nasal Region

Basal cell carcinomas located on the nose, particularly the nasal tip and ala, present unique challenges due to the complex anatomy, the limited availability of surrounding tissues for reconstruction, and the importance of preserving the aesthetic and functional integrity of the nose.

Key management considerations for nasal BCCs include:

1. Careful tumor mapping and delineation: The healthcare provider must accurately map the extent of the tumor, including any subclinical extensions, to ensure complete removal while minimizing the resection of healthy tissue.

2. Specialized surgical techniques: Mohs micrographic surgery is often the preferred surgical approach for nasal BCCs, as it allows for precise margin control and the conservation of healthy tissue, which is crucial for optimal reconstructive outcomes.

3. Reconstructive planning: The healthcare provider, often in collaboration with a plastic surgeon, must carefully plan the reconstruction to achieve the best possible cosmetic and functional results, taking into account the patient's individual anatomy and preferences.

4. Alternative treatment options: In cases where surgical intervention is not feasible or poses a high risk of significant disfigurement, non-surgical approaches, such as radiation therapy or topical medications, may be considered as alternative treatment options.

Auricular Region

Basal cell carcinomas located on the ear, including the pinna, external auditory canal, and surrounding structures, present unique challenges due to the complex three-dimensional anatomy, the potential for involvement of the cartilage and underlying bone, and the importance of preserving hearing function and cosmetic outcomes.

Key management considerations for auricular BCCs include:

1. Comprehensive evaluation: A thorough clinical examination, combined with advanced imaging techniques (e.g., HFUS, CT, MRI), is essential to assess the extent of the tumor and its relationship to critical structures, such as the cartilage, bone, and auditory canal.

2. Specialized surgical techniques: The healthcare provider must employ highly specialized surgical approaches, such as Mohs micrographic surgery or reconstructive techniques involving cartilage or bone grafts, to achieve complete tumor removal while minimizing the impact on hearing and cosmetic outcomes.

3. Multidisciplinary collaboration: The management of auricular BCCs often requires the involvement of dermatologists, otolaryngologists, plastic surgeons, and, in some cases, radiation oncologists, to ensure a comprehensive and coordinated approach to treatment.

4. Alternative treatment modalities: In select cases, where surgical intervention poses a high risk of significant functional or cosmetic impairment, healthcare providers may consider non-surgical options, such as radiation therapy or topical medications, as alternative treatment strategies.

Hereditary Syndromes and Genetic Factors

Certain inherited genetic syndromes are associated with an increased susceptibility to the development of multiple, early-onset basal cell carcinomas. Understanding the unique characteristics and management considerations of these hereditary conditions is crucial for healthcare providers to deliver optimal care to affected patients.

Gorlin Syndrome (Nevoid Basal Cell Carcinoma Syndrome)

Gorlin syndrome, also known as nevoid basal cell carcinoma syndrome (NBCCS), is an autosomal dominant genetic disorder characterized by the development of multiple, recurrent basal cell carcinomas, often at a younger age compared to sporadic BCC cases.

Key features of Gorlin syndrome include:

1. Genetic etiology: Gorlin syndrome is primarily caused by mutations in the PTCH1 gene, a key regulator of the Hedgehog signaling pathway, which plays a central role in the pathogenesis of basal cell carcinoma.

2. Clinical manifestations: In addition to multiple BCCs, individuals with Gorlin syndrome may also develop other characteristic features, such as odontogenic keratocysts, skeletal abnormalities, and an increased risk of certain types of brain tumors (e.g., medulloblastoma).

3. Diagnostic considerations: The diagnosis of Gorlin syndrome is based on a combination of clinical features, family history, and genetic testing. Healthcare providers must maintain a high index of suspicion for this condition, particularly in patients with multiple, early-onset BCCs.

4. Management approach: The management of Gorlin syndrome-associated BCCs requires a comprehensive, multidisciplinary approach, with a focus on early detection, frequent full-body skin examinations, and the implementation of personalized treatment strategies to address the multiplicity and recurrence of these tumors.

5. Targeted therapies: The identification of the underlying genetic basis of Gorlin syndrome has led to the exploration of targeted therapies, such as Hedgehog pathway inhibitors, which may offer a valuable treatment option for these patients.

Other Hereditary Syndromes

While Gorlin syndrome is the most well-known hereditary condition associated with an increased risk of basal cell carcinoma, other rare genetic disorders, such as xeroderma pigmentosum and Bazex-Dupré-Christol syndrome, can also predispose individuals to the development of multiple, early-onset BCCs.

Healthcare providers must be aware of these less common hereditary syndromes and their unique clinical features to ensure timely diagnosis, appropriate genetic testing, and the implementation of personalized management strategies for affected patients.

Immunosuppressed Patients

Individuals with compromised immune systems, such as organ transplant recipients or those undergoing long-term immunosuppressive therapy, face an elevated risk of developing basal cell carcinoma and other non-melanoma skin cancers.

Key Considerations for Immunosuppressed Patients with BCC:

1. Increased incidence and aggressive behavior: Immunosuppressed patients have a significantly higher incidence of BCC, and these tumors may exhibit a more aggressive clinical course, with an increased risk of local invasion, recurrence, and metastasis.

2. Vigilant screening and early detection: Routine full-body skin examinations and a heightened awareness of skin changes are crucial for the early detection of BCCs in immunosuppressed individuals, as these patients may be less able to mount an effective immune response to contain tumor growth.

3. Personalized treatment strategies: The selection of the optimal treatment approach for BCC in immunosuppressed patients must consider the unique challenges posed by their compromised immune status, the potential for

more aggressive tumor behavior, and the impact of any immunosuppressive medications on wound healing and treatment outcomes.

4. Minimizing immunosuppression: In some cases, healthcare providers may explore the possibility of reducing or modifying the immunosuppressive regimen, in collaboration with the patient's transplant or rheumatology team, to mitigate the increased risk of BCC development and recurrence.

5. Heightened surveillance and follow-up: Immunosuppressed patients with BCC require more frequent monitoring and follow-up to detect any signs of recurrence or the development of new lesions, as these individuals are at a higher risk of experiencing multiple primary BCCs over time.

6. Coordination of care: The management of BCC in immunosuppressed patients often requires a multidisciplinary approach, involving dermatologists, oncologists, transplant specialists, and other healthcare providers, to ensure a comprehensive and coordinated plan of care.

Addressing Health Disparities in BCC Management

While the previous sections have highlighted specific clinical scenarios and patient populations that require tailored management approaches, it is crucial to acknowledge the broader issue of health disparities that can impact the care and outcomes of individuals with basal cell carcinoma.

Socioeconomic and Demographic Factors

Factors such as socioeconomic status, race, ethnicity, and geographic location can influence the access to and utilization of healthcare services for BCC diagnosis and treatment. Individuals from underserved or marginalized communities may face barriers in obtaining timely and high-quality skin cancer care, leading to delayed diagnoses, suboptimal treatment, and poorer outcomes.

Healthcare providers and policymakers must prioritize the implementation of strategies to address these disparities, which may include:

1. Improving access to dermatological services: Expanding the availability of specialized care, particularly in underserved areas, through telehealth, mobile clinics, or the integration of skin cancer screening into primary care settings.

2. Enhancing patient education and outreach: Developing culturally appropriate and language-accessible educational materials and campaigns to raise awareness about BCC, skin self-examination, and the importance of seeking timely medical attention.

3. Addressing financial barriers: Implementing policies and programs that improve the affordability and insurance coverage for BCC diagnosis and treatment, particularly for individuals with limited financial resources.

4. Fostering collaborative partnerships: Engaging with community organizations, faith-based groups, and local leaders to build trust, improve outreach, and facilitate access to BCC management services within underserved populations.

5. Promoting diversity and inclusion: Encouraging the recruitment and retention of healthcare providers from diverse backgrounds, who can better understand and address the unique needs of their local communities.

By proactively addressing these health disparities, healthcare providers and policymakers can work towards ensuring equitable access to high-quality basal cell carcinoma care, ultimately improving outcomes and reducing the burden of this disease across all populations.

Conclusion

The management of basal cell carcinoma requires healthcare providers to consider a wide range of special circumstances and unique patient populations. From the challenges posed by BCC lesions in critical anatomical locations to the complexities of hereditary syndromes and immunosuppressed patients, a comprehensive understanding of these special considerations is essential for delivering optimal, personalized care.

By mastering the nuances of BCC management in these specialized clinical scenarios, healthcare providers can ensure that all individuals affected by this common skin cancer receive the most appropriate and effective treatment, tailored to their unique needs and circumstances. This, in turn, can lead to improved patient outcomes, reduced morbidity, and a better overall quality of life.

Furthermore, the recognition and active mitigation of health disparities in BCC care are crucial steps towards promoting equity and ensuring that all members of the community have access to the resources and support necessary for the early detection, prevention, and management of this condition.

The knowledge and insights gained from this chapter will serve as a foundation for the subsequent exploration of the importance of cosmetic and functional outcomes, the role of patient-centered care, and the future directions in the field of basal cell carcinoma management.

CHAPTER 8

Cosmetic and Functional Outcomes

Basal cell carcinoma (BCC) is a common skin cancer that often affects visible and cosmetically sensitive areas of the body, such as the face, head, and neck. While the primary goal of BCC management is to achieve complete tumor removal and disease control, healthcare providers must also prioritize the preservation of aesthetic and functional outcomes for their patients. The potential for scarring, disfigurement, and the impact on quality of life are critical considerations in the comprehensive care of individuals with basal cell carcinoma.

In this chapter, we will explore the strategies and techniques used to optimize cosmetic and functional outcomes in the management of basal cell carcinoma, empowering healthcare providers to deliver personalized, patient-centered care that addresses the multifaceted needs of their patients.

Reconstruction Techniques

The selection of the most appropriate reconstruction technique after the removal of a basal cell carcinoma lesion is a crucial component of the overall treatment plan. Healthcare providers must carefully balance the need for complete tumor removal, the preservation of healthy tissue, and the achievement of the best possible cosmetic and functional outcomes.

Primary Closure

In some cases, particularly for smaller, well-defined BCC lesions, the resulting surgical defect can be closed primarily, with the careful approximation of the wound edges using sutures. This approach aims to minimize the visible scar and maintain the natural contours of the affected area.

However, primary closure may not be suitable for larger defects or in areas where tension on the wound edges could compromise the cosmetic outcome. In these situations, healthcare providers may consider alternative reconstructive techniques.

Skin Grafting

Skin grafting involves the use of a thin layer of skin, harvested from a donor site, to cover the surgical defect left after BCC removal. This technique can be particularly useful for larger defects or in areas where primary closure is not feasible.

The key considerations in skin grafting for BCC reconstruction include:

1. Graft selection: The healthcare provider must carefully select the appropriate type of skin graft, such as a full-thickness or split-thickness graft, based on the size and location of the defect, as well as the desired cosmetic outcome.

2. Donor site selection: The choice of the donor site, such as the behind-the-ear, supraclavicular, or groin areas, can impact the color, texture, and overall appearance of the reconstructed area.

3. Graft placement and fixation: The careful placement and secure fixation of the skin graft are crucial for optimal integration and healing, minimizing the risk of graft failure or contraction.

4. Post-operative management: Proper wound care, dressing changes, and the management of any complications, such as graft loss or infection, are essential for achieving the desired cosmetic outcome.

Flap Reconstruction

Flap reconstruction involves the use of a portion of the patient's own skin and underlying tissue, which is surgically mobilized and rotated or advanced to cover the surgical defect. This technique can be particularly useful for larger defects or in areas where skin grafting may not provide an optimal cosmetic result.

The key advantages of flap reconstruction include the ability to preserve tissue vascularity, maintain the natural contours of the affected area, and potentially achieve a better color and texture match with the surrounding skin.

However, flap reconstruction can be more technically challenging and may require the involvement of a plastic surgeon or a Mohs surgeon with advanced reconstructive expertise. The selection of the appropriate flap design and the execution of the surgical procedure are critical factors in ensuring a successful outcome.

Considerations for Specific Anatomical Locations

The reconstruction of basal cell carcinoma defects in certain anatomical locations, such as the head and neck region, the nose, and the periocular area, requires specialized techniques and a deep understanding of the unique functional and aesthetic considerations.

Head and Neck Region

Basal cell carcinomas located in the head and neck region, particularly on the face, present unique challenges due to the complexity of the anatomy, the presence of critical structures (e.g., eyes, ears, lips), and the high aesthetic importance of this area.

Healthcare providers must carefully plan the reconstruction to minimize scarring, preserve facial symmetry, and maintain important functions, such as vision, speech, and swallowing. Techniques like flap reconstruction, skin grafting, and the use of local tissue rearrangement may be employed to achieve the best possible cosmetic and functional outcomes.

Nose

The reconstruction of BCC defects on the nose, including the nasal tip and ala, is particularly challenging due to the limited availability of surrounding tissues and the importance of maintaining the aesthetic and functional integrity of this prominent facial feature.

Specialized surgical techniques, such as Mohs micrographic surgery followed by the use of nasal subunit reconstruction, can be employed to achieve complete tumor removal while preserving the natural contours and aesthetic appearance of the nose. The involvement of a plastic surgeon or a Mohs surgeon with advanced reconstructive expertise is often crucial in these cases.

Periocular Region

Basal cell carcinomas located in the periocular region, including the eyelids, canthi, and orbital area, require meticulous reconstruction to preserve visual function and maintain a natural, aesthetically pleasing appearance.

The management of periocular BCCs often involves a multidisciplinary approach, with the collaboration of dermatologists, ophthalmologists, and oculoplastic surgeons. Specialized techniques, such as the use of tarsoconjunctival flaps, eyelid-sharing procedures, and the integration of prosthetic or reconstructive materials, may be employed to achieve the desired outcomes.

Minimizing Scarring and Disfigurement

In addition to the reconstruction techniques employed after BCC removal, healthcare providers can also utilize various strategies to minimize the risk of scarring and disfigurement, further enhancing the cosmetic outcomes for their patients.

Surgical Techniques

The selection of the appropriate surgical approach, such as the use of Mohs micrographic surgery or other tissue-sparing techniques, can significantly contribute to the minimization of scarring and disfigurement. These specialized techniques aim to remove the entire tumor while conserving as much healthy tissue as possible, ultimately leading to smaller defects and better cosmetic results.

Furthermore, the careful execution of the surgical procedure, including the precise placement of incisions, the meticulous handling of tissues, and the use of fine suturing techniques, can help reduce the visibility and appearance of scars.

Wound Care and Scar Management

Proper wound care and the implementation of evidence-based scar management strategies can also play a crucial role in minimizing the appearance of scars after BCC removal.

Healthcare providers may recommend the use of specialized dressings, topical scar treatments, and even the application of silicone-based products to help flatten, soften, and fade the appearance of scars. Additionally, the timely initiation of scar massage and other physical therapy interventions can improve the overall cosmetic outcome.

In some cases, the use of laser therapy or other resurfacing techniques may be considered to further enhance the appearance of scars, particularly in cases where significant scarring is unavoidable.

Psychological and Emotional Impact

The potential for scarring, disfigurement, and the impact on physical appearance can have a significant psychological and emotional impact on individuals with basal cell carcinoma. Healthcare providers must be attuned to these concerns and incorporate strategies to address the patient's emotional well-being as an integral part of the comprehensive management approach.

Addressing Psychological Distress

Healthcare providers should actively screen for and address any signs of psychological distress, such as anxiety, depression, or body image concerns, that may arise in patients with BCC. This may involve the integration of psychological counseling, support groups, or referrals to mental health professionals as part of the overall care plan.

Furthermore, healthcare providers can empower patients by educating them about the various reconstructive options and scar management strategies available, helping to set realistic expectations and alleviate concerns about the potential cosmetic outcomes.

Fostering Resilience and Coping Strategies

In addition to addressing psychological distress, healthcare providers can also work with patients to foster resilience and develop effective coping strategies. Techniques such as mindfulness, stress management, and the cultivation of a positive self-image can help individuals with BCC navigate the emotional challenges associated with the condition and its treatment.

By incorporating these psychosocial interventions into the comprehensive management of basal cell carcinoma, healthcare providers can ensure that the care they provide addresses the holistic needs of their patients, ultimately improving their overall quality of life.

Improving Quality of Life

The primary goal of basal cell carcinoma management is to achieve complete tumor removal and disease control. However, it is equally important to prioritize the enhancement of the patient's quality of life, which can be significantly impacted by the cosmetic and functional outcomes of the treatment.

Shared Decision-Making

Healthcare providers should engage in a collaborative, shared decision-making process with their patients to ensure that the selected treatment approach aligns with the patient's individual goals, preferences, and expectations. This may involve discussing the various surgical and non-surgical options, the anticipated cosmetic outcomes, and the potential impact on the patient's daily activities and well-being.

By involving the patient in the decision-making process, healthcare providers can foster a sense of empowerment and facilitate the development of a personalized care plan that optimizes both the clinical and quality-of-life outcomes.

Patient-Reported Outcomes

The incorporation of patient-reported outcome measures (PROMs) can provide valuable insights into the patient's experience and the impact of the chosen treatment on their quality of life. PROMs may include assessments of symptom burden, functional status, cosmetic satisfaction, and overall well-being.

The systematic collection and analysis of PROM data can help healthcare providers identify areas for improvement, tailor their interventions to better meet the patient's needs, and track the long-term impact of the treatment on the patient's quality of life.

Interdisciplinary Collaboration

Achieving optimal cosmetic and functional outcomes for individuals with basal cell carcinoma often requires the expertise and collaboration of various healthcare providers, including dermatologists, plastic surgeons, oculoplastic surgeons, and rehabilitation specialists.

By fostering an interdisciplinary approach, healthcare providers can leverage their collective knowledge and skills to develop a comprehensive treatment plan that addresses the unique needs of each patient, maximizing the chances of achieving the desired cosmetic and functional results.

Conclusion

The management of basal cell carcinoma must extend beyond the mere removal of the tumor and consider the preservation of cosmetic and functional outcomes as an integral part of the comprehensive care plan. Healthcare providers must prioritize the use of specialized reconstruction techniques, the minimization of scarring and disfigurement, and the incorporation of psychosocial interventions to address the holistic needs of their patients.

By adopting a patient-centered approach that emphasizes shared decision-making, the integration of patient-reported outcomes, and the collaboration of an interdisciplinary team, healthcare providers can ensure that the care they provide for individuals with basal cell carcinoma not only achieves disease control but also enhances the patient's overall quality of life.

The knowledge and insights gained from this chapter will serve as a foundation for the subsequent exploration of the importance of long-term follow-up and survivorship care, the role of integrated and complementary approaches, and the ongoing advancements in the field of basal cell carcinoma management.

CHAPTER 9

Integrative and Complementary Approaches

As the comprehensive management of basal cell carcinoma (BCC) continues to evolve, healthcare providers and patients have increasingly explored the potential role of integrative and complementary approaches in the holistic care of this common skin cancer. While traditional medical interventions, such as surgical and non-surgical treatments, remain the foundation of BCC management, the integration of evidence-based complementary therapies can provide a valuable addition to the overall care plan, addressing the multifaceted needs of individuals affected by this condition.

In this chapter, we will delve into the potential benefits and considerations of incorporating integrative and complementary approaches into the management of basal cell carcinoma, empowering healthcare providers and patients to make informed decisions and adopt a more holistic approach to their care.

Dietary and Lifestyle Modifications

The role of dietary and lifestyle modifications in the prevention and management of basal cell carcinoma has been the subject of ongoing research and growing interest among healthcare providers and patients.

Dietary Factors

Several studies have suggested that certain dietary components may play a role in the prevention and potentially the management of basal cell carcinoma.

1. Carotenoids: Dietary carotenoids, such as beta-carotene and lycopene, have been associated with a reduced risk of developing BCC, potentially due to their antioxidant and photoprotective properties.

2. Vitamins and minerals: Adequate intake of vitamins C, E, and selenium, as well as the mineral zinc, have been linked to a decreased incidence of basal cell carcinoma in some studies.

3. Omega-3 fatty acids: The anti-inflammatory properties of omega-3 fatty acids, found in foods like fatty fish, walnuts, and flaxseeds, may provide some protective benefits against BCC development.

4. Plant-based compounds: Certain phytochemicals, such as resveratrol, curcumin, and green tea polyphenols, have demonstrated potential anti-cancer and chemopreventive effects in preclinical studies, suggesting a possible role in BCC management.

Healthcare providers should educate patients on the potential benefits of incorporating these dietary components into their daily lives, while also emphasizing the importance of maintaining a balanced and nutrient-rich diet.

Lifestyle Modifications

In addition to dietary factors, specific lifestyle modifications may also contribute to the prevention and management of basal cell carcinoma.

1. Sun exposure and UV protection: As discussed in previous chapters, the avoidance of excessive sun exposure and the consistent use of sun-protective

measures, such as sunscreen, protective clothing, and limiting the use of tanning beds, are crucial for reducing the risk of developing new or recurrent BCC lesions.

2. Smoking cessation: Cigarette smoking has been associated with an increased risk of developing basal cell carcinoma, particularly in older individuals. Healthcare providers should encourage patients to quit smoking and provide access to appropriate cessation resources.

3. Stress management: Chronic stress has been linked to various health problems, including a potential increased risk of skin cancer. Incorporating stress-reducing techniques, such as mindfulness, meditation, or regular exercise, may be beneficial for BCC patients.

4. Physical activity: Regular physical activity has been associated with a reduced risk of developing basal cell carcinoma, potentially due to its anti-inflammatory effects and impact on the immune system.

By empowering patients to adopt these evidence-based dietary and lifestyle modifications, healthcare providers can empower individuals to take an active role in their skin health and potentially contribute to the prevention and management of basal cell carcinoma.

Stress Management and Relaxation Techniques

The diagnosis and management of basal cell carcinoma can be a significant source of stress and psychological distress for patients, as discussed in previous chapters. Incorporating stress management and relaxation techniques into the comprehensive care plan can provide a valuable complement to the traditional medical interventions.

Mindfulness and Meditation

Mindfulness-based practices, such as mindfulness meditation, have been studied for their potential benefits in reducing stress, anxiety, and depression in individuals with various health conditions, including skin cancer.

The practice of mindfulness involves the cultivation of present-moment awareness, self-compassion, and the ability to manage negative thoughts and emotions. By integrating mindfulness-based techniques into their daily lives, BCC patients may experience improved coping mechanisms, reduced psychological distress, and enhanced overall well-being.

Healthcare providers can encourage their patients to explore mindfulness-based approaches, such as guided meditations, body scans, or mindful breathing exercises, and provide resources for learning and practicing these techniques.

Relaxation Techniques

In addition to mindfulness-based practices, healthcare providers may also recommend various relaxation techniques to help BCC patients manage stress and promote overall well-being.

These techniques may include:

1. Progressive muscle relaxation: This involves the systematic tensing and relaxing of different muscle groups to induce a state of physical and mental calmness.

2. Deep breathing exercises: Controlled, deep breathing patterns can help activate the parasympathetic nervous system, promoting a relaxation response.

3. Visualization and imagery: Guided visualizations or imagining peaceful, soothing scenes can help reduce anxiety and promote a sense of calm.

4. Yoga and tai chi: These mind-body practices combine physical movements, breathing, and meditation, offering a holistic approach to stress management.

By incorporating these relaxation techniques into the comprehensive care of basal cell carcinoma patients, healthcare providers can empower individuals to develop effective coping strategies and enhance their overall quality of life throughout the management of their condition.

Evidence-Based Complementary Therapies

While dietary and lifestyle modifications, as well as stress management techniques, can provide a valuable complement to traditional medical interventions, there are also several other complementary therapies that have been explored for their potential benefits in the management of basal cell carcinoma.

Topical Herbal Treatments

Several herbal and plant-based compounds have been investigated for their potential efficacy in the topical treatment of basal cell carcinoma. These include:

1. Betulinic acid: Derived from the bark of the birch tree, betulinic acid has demonstrated anti-tumor and pro-apoptotic effects in preclinical studies, suggesting a possible role in BCC management.

2. Curcumin: The active compound in turmeric, curcumin, has been studied for its anti-inflammatory and anti-cancer properties, with some evidence suggesting a potential benefit in the treatment of BCC.

3. Green tea polyphenols: The polyphenols found in green tea, particularly epigallocatechin gallate (EGCG), have shown promise in preclinical studies for their ability to inhibit the growth and proliferation of BCC cells.

While these topical herbal treatments are not currently approved for the primary treatment of basal cell carcinoma, some healthcare providers may consider them as adjuncts or alternatives for select patients, particularly those who are unable or unwilling to undergo conventional surgical or non-surgical interventions.

It is important to note that the use of these complementary therapies should be discussed with the healthcare provider, as their safety, efficacy, and potential interactions with conventional treatments must be carefully evaluated.

Photodynamic Therapy

Photodynamic therapy (PDT), as discussed in Chapter 5, is a non-surgical treatment approach that utilizes the combination of a photosensitizing agent and targeted light exposure to selectively destroy basal cell carcinoma tumor cells. While PDT is considered a conventional non-surgical treatment option, it can also be viewed as a complementary approach that integrates the use of light-based therapy with the body's natural mechanisms of tumor destruction.

The advantages of photodynamic therapy as a complementary approach to BCC management include its non-invasive nature, the potential for improved cosmetic outcomes, and the ability to treat multiple lesions simultaneously. Furthermore, PDT has been shown to have an excellent safety profile, with a relatively low risk of long-term adverse effects.

Healthcare providers may consider incorporating photodynamic therapy into the comprehensive management of basal cell carcinoma, particularly for select patients who are not suitable candidates for or have a preference against more invasive surgical or non-surgical interventions.

Acupuncture and Traditional Chinese Medicine

The use of acupuncture and traditional Chinese medicine (TCM) has been explored as a potential complementary approach in the management of various skin conditions, including basal cell carcinoma.

While the scientific evidence for the effectiveness of acupuncture and TCM in the primary treatment of BCC is limited, some studies have suggested potential benefits in the alleviation of treatment-related side effects, the management of pain and other symptoms, and the improvement of overall well-being for individuals with this condition.

Healthcare providers should be aware of the availability of these complementary therapies and be prepared to discuss their potential role, limitations, and any known interactions with their patients. Collaboration with qualified acupuncturists or TCM practitioners can help ensure the safe and appropriate integration of these modalities into the comprehensive care plan for basal cell carcinoma.

Patient Education and Shared Decision-Making

The incorporation of integrative and complementary approaches into the management of basal cell carcinoma must be grounded in a collaborative, patient-centered approach that emphasizes education and shared decision-making between healthcare providers and their patients.

Patient Education

Educating patients about the potential role of integrative and complementary therapies in the management of BCC is crucial. Healthcare providers should:

1. Provide evidence-based information about the available complementary options, their potential benefits, and any known limitations or risks.
2. Encourage patients to discuss their interest in or use of complementary

therapies openly and without judgment.

3. Ensure that patients understand the importance of maintaining open communication with their healthcare team regarding the use of any complementary modalities.

By empowering patients with knowledge and fostering a culture of transparency, healthcare providers can help individuals make informed decisions about the integration of complementary approaches into their comprehensive BCC care plan.

Shared Decision-Making

The selection and integration of integrative and complementary therapies should be a collaborative process between the healthcare provider and the patient. Healthcare providers should:

1. Actively solicit the patient's preferences, concerns, and goals regarding the use of complementary approaches.
2. Discuss the potential benefits, limitations, and risks of incorporating specific complementary modalities into the overall care plan.
3. Work with the patient to develop a personalized, integrative care plan that aligns with the patient's values, resources, and individual needs.

By embracing a shared decision-making approach, healthcare providers can empower patients to take an active role in their care, fostering a sense of engagement and ownership over the management of their basal cell carcinoma.

Multidisciplinary Collaboration

The successful integration of integrative and complementary approaches into the care of basal cell carcinoma patients often requires a multidisciplinary collaboration among various healthcare providers, including dermatologists, primary care physicians, oncologists, nutritionists, mental health professionals, and complementary and alternative medicine practitioners.

This interdisciplinary team can work together to:

1. Develop evidence-based guidelines and protocols for the safe and effective integration of complementary therapies into BCC management.
2. Facilitate the coordination of care, ensuring seamless communication and the alignment of the patient's overall treatment plan.
3. Provide comprehensive patient education and support, empowering individuals to make informed decisions about the use of integrative approaches.
4. Monitor the patient's progress and response to the integrated care plan, making necessary adjustments to optimize outcomes.

By fostering this collaborative, multidisciplinary approach, healthcare providers can ensure that the integration of complementary therapies into the management of basal cell carcinoma is well-coordinated, evidence-based, and truly patient-centered.

Conclusion

The incorporation of integrative and complementary approaches into the comprehensive management of basal cell carcinoma can provide a valuable complement to traditional medical interventions. By exploring the potential benefits of dietary and lifestyle modifications, stress management techniques, and select evidence-based complementary therapies, healthcare providers can empower their patients to take a more active role in their skin health and overall well-being.

However, the integration of these complementary modalities must be grounded in a collaborative, patient-centered approach that emphasizes education, shared decision-making, and multidisciplinary coordination. By adopting this holistic perspective, healthcare providers can deliver personalized, integrative care that addresses the multifaceted needs of individuals affected by basal cell carcinoma.

The knowledge and insights gained from this chapter will serve as a foundation for the subsequent exploration of global perspectives and health disparities in BCC management, as well as the ongoing research and innovations that are shaping the future of this field.

CHAPTER 10

Integrative and Complementary Approaches

As the comprehensive management of basal cell carcinoma (BCC) continues to evolve, healthcare providers and patients have increasingly explored the potential role of integrative and complementary approaches in the holistic care of this common skin cancer. While traditional medical interventions, such as surgical and non-surgical treatments, remain the foundation of BCC management, the integration of evidence-based complementary therapies can provide a valuable addition to the overall care plan, addressing the multifaceted needs of individuals affected by this condition.

In this chapter, we will delve into the potential benefits and considerations of incorporating integrative and complementary approaches into the management of basal cell carcinoma, empowering healthcare providers and patients to make informed decisions and adopt a more holistic approach to their care.

Dietary and Lifestyle Modifications

The role of dietary and lifestyle modifications in the prevention and management of basal cell carcinoma has been the subject of ongoing research and growing interest among healthcare providers and patients.

Dietary Factors

Several studies have suggested that certain dietary components may play a role in the prevention and potentially the management of basal cell carcinoma.

1. Carotenoids: Dietary carotenoids, such as beta-carotene and lycopene, have been associated with a reduced risk of developing BCC, potentially due to their antioxidant and photoprotective properties.

2. Vitamins and minerals: Adequate intake of vitamins C, E, and selenium, as well as the mineral zinc, have been linked to a decreased incidence of basal cell carcinoma in some studies.

3. Omega-3 fatty acids: The anti-inflammatory properties of omega-3 fatty acids, found in foods like fatty fish, walnuts, and flaxseeds, may provide some protective benefits against BCC development.

4. Plant-based compounds: Certain phytochemicals, such as resveratrol, curcumin, and green tea polyphenols, have demonstrated potential anti-cancer and chemopreventive effects in preclinical studies, suggesting a possible role in BCC management.

Healthcare providers should educate patients on the potential benefits of incorporating these dietary components into their daily lives, while also emphasizing the importance of maintaining a balanced and nutrient-rich diet.

Lifestyle Modifications

In addition to dietary factors, specific lifestyle modifications may also contribute to the prevention and management of basal cell carcinoma.

1. Sun exposure and UV protection: As discussed in previous chapters, the avoidance of excessive sun exposure and the consistent use of sun-protective

measures, such as sunscreen, protective clothing, and limiting the use of tanning beds, are crucial for reducing the risk of developing new or recurrent BCC lesions.

2. Smoking cessation: Cigarette smoking has been associated with an increased risk of developing basal cell carcinoma, particularly in older individuals. Healthcare providers should encourage patients to quit smoking and provide access to appropriate cessation resources.

3. Stress management: Chronic stress has been linked to various health problems, including a potential increased risk of skin cancer. Incorporating stress-reducing techniques, such as mindfulness, meditation, or regular exercise, may be beneficial for BCC patients.

4. Physical activity: Regular physical activity has been associated with a reduced risk of developing basal cell carcinoma, potentially due to its anti-inflammatory effects and impact on the immune system.

By empowering patients to adopt these evidence-based dietary and lifestyle modifications, healthcare providers can empower individuals to take an active role in their skin health and potentially contribute to the prevention and management of basal cell carcinoma.

Stress Management and Relaxation Techniques

The diagnosis and management of basal cell carcinoma can be a significant source of stress and psychological distress for patients, as discussed in previous chapters. Incorporating stress management and relaxation techniques into the comprehensive care plan can provide a valuable complement to the traditional medical interventions.

Mindfulness and Meditation

Mindfulness-based practices, such as mindfulness meditation, have been studied for their potential benefits in reducing stress, anxiety, and depression in individuals with various health conditions, including skin cancer.

The practice of mindfulness involves the cultivation of present-moment awareness, self-compassion, and the ability to manage negative thoughts and emotions. By integrating mindfulness-based techniques into their daily lives, BCC patients may experience improved coping mechanisms, reduced psychological distress, and enhanced overall well-being.

Healthcare providers can encourage their patients to explore mindfulness-based approaches, such as guided meditations, body scans, or mindful breathing exercises, and provide resources for learning and practicing these techniques.

Relaxation Techniques

In addition to mindfulness-based practices, healthcare providers may also recommend various relaxation techniques to help BCC patients manage stress and promote overall well-being.

These techniques may include:

1. Progressive muscle relaxation: This involves the systematic tensing and relaxing of different muscle groups to induce a state of physical and mental calmness.

2. Deep breathing exercises: Controlled, deep breathing patterns can help activate the parasympathetic nervous system, promoting a relaxation response.

3. Visualization and imagery: Guided visualizations or imagining peaceful, soothing scenes can help reduce anxiety and promote a sense of calm.

4. Yoga and tai chi: These mind-body practices combine physical movements, breathing, and meditation, offering a holistic approach to stress management.

By incorporating these relaxation techniques into the comprehensive care of basal cell carcinoma patients, healthcare providers can empower individuals to develop effective coping strategies and enhance their overall quality of life throughout the management of their condition.

Evidence-Based Complementary Therapies

While dietary and lifestyle modifications, as well as stress management techniques, can provide a valuable complement to traditional medical interventions, there are also several other complementary therapies that have been explored for their potential benefits in the management of basal cell carcinoma.

Topical Herbal Treatments

Several herbal and plant-based compounds have been investigated for their potential efficacy in the topical treatment of basal cell carcinoma. These include:

1. Betulinic acid: Derived from the bark of the birch tree, betulinic acid has demonstrated anti-tumor and pro-apoptotic effects in preclinical studies, suggesting a possible role in BCC management.

2. Curcumin: The active compound in turmeric, curcumin, has been studied for its anti-inflammatory and anti-cancer properties, with some evidence suggesting a potential benefit in the treatment of BCC.

3. Green tea polyphenols: The polyphenols found in green tea, particularly epigallocatechin gallate (EGCG), have shown promise in preclinical studies for their ability to inhibit the growth and proliferation of BCC cells.

While these topical herbal treatments are not currently approved for the primary treatment of basal cell carcinoma, some healthcare providers may consider them as adjuncts or alternatives for select patients, particularly those who are unable or unwilling to undergo conventional surgical or non-surgical interventions.

It is important to note that the use of these complementary therapies should be discussed with the healthcare provider, as their safety, efficacy, and potential interactions with conventional treatments must be carefully evaluated.

Photodynamic Therapy

Photodynamic therapy (PDT), as discussed in Chapter 5, is a non-surgical treatment approach that utilizes the combination of a photosensitizing agent and targeted light exposure to selectively destroy basal cell carcinoma tumor cells. While PDT is considered a conventional non-surgical treatment option, it can also be viewed as a complementary approach that integrates the use of light-based therapy with the body's natural mechanisms of tumor destruction.

The advantages of photodynamic therapy as a complementary approach to BCC management include its non-invasive nature, the potential for improved cosmetic outcomes, and the ability to treat multiple lesions simultaneously. Furthermore, PDT has been shown to have an excellent safety profile, with a relatively low risk of long-term adverse effects.

Healthcare providers may consider incorporating photodynamic therapy into the comprehensive management of basal cell carcinoma, particularly for select patients who are not suitable candidates for or have a preference against more invasive surgical or non-surgical interventions.

Acupuncture and Traditional Chinese Medicine

The use of acupuncture and traditional Chinese medicine (TCM) has been explored as a potential complementary approach in the management of various skin conditions, including basal cell carcinoma.

While the scientific evidence for the effectiveness of acupuncture and TCM in the primary treatment of BCC is limited, some studies have suggested potential benefits in the alleviation of treatment-related side effects, the management of pain and other symptoms, and the improvement of overall well-being for individuals with this condition.

Healthcare providers should be aware of the availability of these complementary therapies and be prepared to discuss their potential role, limitations, and any known interactions with their patients. Collaboration with qualified acupuncturists or TCM practitioners can help ensure the safe and appropriate integration of these modalities into the comprehensive care plan for basal cell carcinoma.

Patient Education and Shared Decision-Making

The incorporation of integrative and complementary approaches into the management of basal cell carcinoma must be grounded in a collaborative, patient-centered approach that emphasizes education and shared decision-making between healthcare providers and their patients.

Patient Education

Educating patients about the potential role of integrative and complementary therapies in the management of BCC is crucial. Healthcare providers should:

1. Provide evidence-based information about the available complementary options, their potential benefits, and any known limitations or risks.
2. Encourage patients to discuss their interest in or use of complementary

therapies openly and without judgment.

3. Ensure that patients understand the importance of maintaining open communication with their healthcare team regarding the use of any complementary modalities.

By empowering patients with knowledge and fostering a culture of transparency, healthcare providers can help individuals make informed decisions about the integration of complementary approaches into their comprehensive BCC care plan.

Shared Decision-Making

The selection and integration of integrative and complementary therapies should be a collaborative process between the healthcare provider and the patient. Healthcare providers should:

1. Actively solicit the patient's preferences, concerns, and goals regarding the use of complementary approaches.
2. Discuss the potential benefits, limitations, and risks of incorporating specific complementary modalities into the overall care plan.
3. Work with the patient to develop a personalized, integrative care plan that aligns with the patient's values, resources, and individual needs.

By embracing a shared decision-making approach, healthcare providers can empower patients to take an active role in their care, fostering a sense of engagement and ownership over the management of their basal cell carcinoma.

Multidisciplinary Collaboration

The successful integration of integrative and complementary approaches into the care of basal cell carcinoma patients often requires a multidisciplinary collaboration among various healthcare providers, including dermatologists, primary care physicians, oncologists, nutritionists, mental health professionals, and complementary and alternative medicine practitioners.

This interdisciplinary team can work together to:

1. Develop evidence-based guidelines and protocols for the safe and effective integration of complementary therapies into BCC management.
2. Facilitate the coordination of care, ensuring seamless communication and the alignment of the patient's overall treatment plan.
3. Provide comprehensive patient education and support, empowering individuals to make informed decisions about the use of integrative approaches.
4. Monitor the patient's progress and response to the integrated care plan, making necessary adjustments to optimize outcomes.

By fostering this collaborative, multidisciplinary approach, healthcare providers can ensure that the integration of complementary therapies into the management of basal cell carcinoma is well-coordinated, evidence-based, and truly patient-centered.

Conclusion

The incorporation of integrative and complementary approaches into the comprehensive management of basal cell carcinoma can provide a valuable complement to traditional medical interventions. By exploring the potential benefits of dietary and lifestyle modifications, stress management techniques, and select evidence-based complementary therapies, healthcare providers can empower their patients to take a more active role in their skin health and overall well-being.

However, the integration of these complementary modalities must be grounded in a collaborative, patient-centered approach that emphasizes education, shared decision-making, and multidisciplinary coordination. By adopting this holistic perspective, healthcare providers can deliver personalized, integrative care that addresses the multifaceted needs of individuals affected by basal cell carcinoma.

The knowledge and insights gained from this chapter will serve as a foundation for the subsequent exploration of global perspectives and health disparities in BCC management, as well as the ongoing research and innovations that are shaping the future of this field.

CHAPTER 11

Global Perspectives and Health Disparities

Basal cell carcinoma (BCC) is a global health concern, with its incidence and management varying across different geographic regions and populations. Understanding the nuances of basal cell carcinoma from an international perspective is crucial, as it can inform healthcare policies, guide the development of tailored interventions, and promote more equitable access to care for individuals affected by this common skin cancer.

In this chapter, we will explore the global landscape of basal cell carcinoma, examining the variations in incidence, management strategies, and the challenges of addressing health disparities in the diagnosis and treatment of this condition.

Global Epidemiology and Incidence Trends

Basal cell carcinoma is the most common form of skin cancer worldwide, with its incidence continuing to rise in many parts of the globe. However, the epidemiological patterns and trends of BCC can vary significantly across different regions and populations.

Geographic Variations

The incidence of basal cell carcinoma is highest in countries with predominantly fair-skinned populations and a high level of ultraviolet (UV) radiation exposure, such as Australia, New Zealand, and certain parts of the United States and Europe. In these regions, BCC often accounts for a significant proportion of all skin cancer diagnoses.

In contrast, the reported incidence of basal cell carcinoma is generally lower in countries with predominantly darker-skinned populations, such as many African and Asian nations. This variation can be attributed to factors like differences in skin pigmentation, sun exposure patterns, and potentially genetic predispositions.

It is important to note that the apparent lower incidence of BCC in certain regions may also be influenced by underreporting, limited access to healthcare, or differences in diagnostic practices and disease surveillance systems.

Temporal Trends

Over the past several decades, the global incidence of basal cell carcinoma has been steadily increasing, driven by a combination of factors, including:

1. Increased UV exposure: Changes in lifestyle and leisure activities, such as the growing popularity of outdoor recreation and the use of tanning beds, have contributed to the rise in UV exposure among the general population.

2. Aging population: As the global population ages, the number of individuals at risk for developing basal cell carcinoma has increased, as the incidence of BCC tends to rise with advancing age.

3. Improved disease detection: Advances in diagnostic techniques and increased awareness among healthcare providers and the general public have led to the improved detection and reporting of BCC cases.

Understanding these global epidemiological trends is crucial for healthcare providers and policymakers to anticipate the future burden of basal cell carcinoma, allocate appropriate resources, and develop tailored strategies for prevention and management.

Variations in Management Strategies

The approach to the management of basal cell carcinoma can vary significantly across different healthcare systems and geographic regions, reflecting differences in resource availability, healthcare infrastructure, cultural preferences, and evidence-based guidelines.

Surgical Interventions

In many high-income countries, surgical interventions, such as Mohs micrographic surgery and standard surgical excision, are often the preferred treatment modalities for basal cell carcinoma. These specialized techniques are widely available and have been adopted as the standard of care in these settings.

However, in resource-limited or underserved regions, access to specialized surgical services may be more limited, leading to a greater reliance on alternative treatment approaches, such as cryotherapy, curettage, or even less sophisticated surgical methods.

The availability and utilization of these specialized surgical techniques can have a significant impact on patient outcomes, as they are generally associated with higher cure rates and better cosmetic results compared to some of the more basic surgical approaches.

Non-Surgical Interventions

The accessibility and implementation of non-surgical treatment options for basal cell carcinoma, such as topical medications, photodynamic therapy, and radiation therapy, can also vary considerably across different healthcare systems and regions.

In some high-income countries, these non-surgical modalities may be readily available and integrated into the standard of care for BCC management. In contrast, in resource-constrained settings, the use of these treatments may be more limited due to factors such as the availability of specialized equipment, the cost of the therapies, and the expertise required for their administration.

The disparities in access to non-surgical interventions can have a significant impact on patient outcomes, particularly for individuals who may not be suitable candidates for or prefer to avoid surgical treatments.

Systemic Therapies

The availability and utilization of systemic therapies, specifically targeted Hedgehog pathway inhibitors, for the management of advanced or metastatic basal cell carcinoma can also vary globally.

These innovative targeted agents have revolutionized the care of high-risk BCC cases in many high-income countries, where they are approved and accessible. However, in resource-limited settings or regions with limited healthcare infrastructure, the availability and affordability of these specialized systemic therapies may be more restricted, leaving patients with fewer treatment options for advanced or aggressive forms of the disease.

The disparities in access to cutting-edge systemic therapies can contribute to disparities in overall disease outcomes and quality of life for individuals with high-risk or advanced basal cell carcinoma.

Addressing Health Disparities in BCC Care

The variations in the incidence, management strategies, and access to care for basal cell carcinoma across different geographic regions and populations highlight the critical need to address health disparities in the diagnosis, treatment, and long-term management of this common skin cancer.

Improving Access to Dermatological Services

One of the key strategies for addressing health disparities in basal cell carcinoma care is to improve access to specialized dermatological services, particularly in underserved or resource-limited areas.

This may involve:

1. Expanding the availability of dermatologists and trained healthcare providers: Initiatives to incentivize the recruitment and retention of dermatologists in underserved regions can help bridge the gap in access to specialized care.

2. Integrating skin cancer screening and management into primary care: Empowering primary care providers to incorporate routine skin examinations and the initial management of BCC into their scope of practice can enhance the accessibility of care, especially in areas with limited access to dermatologists.

3. Leveraging telemedicine and digital health technologies: The use of telehealth and mobile health applications can facilitate the remote delivery of dermatological services, improving access to specialized care for individuals in geographically remote or underserved areas.

4. Establishing mobile skin cancer clinics: Deploying mobile screening and treatment units to underserved communities can help reach individuals who may face barriers to accessing traditional healthcare facilities.

Enhancing Patient Education and Outreach

Improving patient education and outreach efforts is another crucial component in addressing health disparities in basal cell carcinoma care. This may include:

1. Developing culturally appropriate and linguistically accessible educational materials: Ensuring that patient education resources are tailored to the specific cultural and language needs of diverse populations can enhance their effectiveness and uptake.

2. Partnering with community organizations and leaders: Collaborating with local community-based organizations, faith-based groups, and trusted community leaders can help build trust, raise awareness, and facilitate access to BCC screening and management services.

3. Implementing targeted public health campaigns: Focused public health initiatives that raise awareness about the importance of skin cancer prevention, early detection, and access to care can help address disparities in BCC knowledge and healthcare-seeking behaviors.

4. Promoting skin self-examination and empowering patients: Educating individuals on the importance of regular skin self-examinations and providing the necessary tools and resources can empower them to take an active role in their skin health.

Addressing Financial Barriers to Care

Financial barriers, such as the cost of diagnosis, treatment, and follow-up care, can significantly impact access to basal cell carcinoma management, particularly for individuals from low-income or underinsured backgrounds.

Strategies to address these financial barriers may include:

1. Implementing universal healthcare coverage or expanding insurance programs: Ensuring that comprehensive skin cancer care is included in the benefits package of public or private insurance programs can improve affordability and access to BCC management.

2. Establishing patient assistance programs: Developing programs that provide financial support, such as subsidies or discounts, for individuals who cannot afford the cost of BCC diagnosis and treatment can help overcome economic barriers to care.

3. Advocating for policy changes and increased funding: Engaging with policymakers and advocating for the allocation of resources to support comprehensive skin cancer prevention and management initiatives can help address the systemic barriers to equitable access.

Fostering Diversity and Inclusion in the Healthcare Workforce

The diversity and representation of healthcare providers, particularly dermatologists and other specialists involved in the management of basal cell carcinoma, can have a significant impact on addressing health disparities and providing culturally competent care.

Strategies to promote diversity and inclusion in the healthcare workforce may include:

1. Targeted recruitment and mentorship programs: Initiatives that encourage and support the recruitment and retention of healthcare providers from diverse backgrounds can help improve the representation of underserved populations in the field of dermatology and skin cancer care.

2. Culturally competent training and education: Incorporating cultural competency and implicit bias training into the curricula of medical and healthcare professional programs can enhance the ability of providers to

deliver more inclusive and patient-centered care.

3. Promoting community engagement and outreach: Encouraging healthcare providers to engage with local communities, participate in outreach events, and build trust-based relationships can foster a more equitable and accessible healthcare system for individuals affected by basal cell carcinoma.

By addressing these multifaceted barriers to care and promoting inclusive, patient-centered approaches, healthcare systems and policymakers can work towards ensuring that all individuals affected by basal cell carcinoma have access to high-quality, evidence-based care, regardless of their geographic location or socioeconomic status.

Global Collaborations and Knowledge Sharing

In the pursuit of addressing health disparities and improving the management of basal cell carcinoma on a global scale, collaborative efforts and the sharing of knowledge and best practices among healthcare providers, researchers, and policymakers across different regions are essential.

International Skin Cancer Registries and Databases

The establishment of comprehensive, multinational skin cancer registries and databases can play a crucial role in enhancing our understanding of the global epidemiology, management strategies, and outcomes associated with basal cell carcinoma.

These collaborative efforts can:

1. Facilitate the collection and aggregation of standardized data on BCC incidence, treatment approaches, and long-term outcomes across diverse populations and healthcare settings.

2. Enable the identification of geographic and demographic variations in BCC management and disease burden, informing the development of targeted interventions and resource allocation.
3. Promote the sharing of best practices, evidence-based guidelines, and innovative strategies for addressing health disparities in skin cancer care.

By fostering international collaborations and the exchange of knowledge through these comprehensive data platforms, healthcare providers and policymakers can work towards improving the global management of basal cell carcinoma and ensuring more equitable access to high-quality care.

Global Guidelines and Standards of Care

The development and dissemination of evidence-based, globally harmonized guidelines and standards of care for the management of basal cell carcinoma can also play a crucial role in addressing health disparities and promoting consistent, high-quality care across different regions.

These global guidelines can:

1. Establish standardized diagnostic and treatment protocols that can be adapted and implemented in diverse healthcare settings.
2. Provide recommendations for the integration of novel therapies, such as targeted systemic treatments, into the comprehensive management of BCC, ensuring timely access to cutting-edge interventions.
3. Offer guidance on the implementation of cost-effective, scalable strategies for skin cancer prevention, early detection, and long-term follow-up, particularly in resource-limited settings.

By aligning healthcare providers and policymakers around a common, evidence-based framework for basal cell carcinoma management, these global guidelines can help bridge the gaps in care and promote more equitable access to high-quality skin cancer services worldwide.

Conclusion

Basal cell carcinoma is a global health concern, with its incidence, management strategies, and access to care varying significantly across different geographic regions and populations. Understanding these global perspectives and addressing the health disparities associated with BCC are crucial steps towards ensuring that all individuals affected by this common skin cancer receive the comprehensive, patient-centered care they deserve.

By improving access to dermatological services, enhancing patient education and outreach, addressing financial barriers to care, and fostering diversity and inclusion in the healthcare workforce, healthcare systems and policymakers can work towards mitigating the disparities in basal cell carcinoma management. Furthermore, the establishment of global collaborations, international registries, and harmonized guidelines can facilitate the sharing of knowledge and the implementation of best practices, ultimately improving outcomes for individuals affected by BCC worldwide.

The insights and strategies discussed in this chapter will serve as a foundation for the subsequent exploration of the future directions and research priorities in the field of basal cell carcinoma management, as we strive to continually enhance the care and well-being of all patients affected by this prevalent skin malignancy.

CHAPTER 12

C hapter 12: Future Directions and Research Priorities

As the landscape of basal cell carcinoma (BCC) management continues to evolve, healthcare providers and researchers are constantly exploring new frontiers, seeking to enhance diagnostic capabilities, improve treatment strategies, and ultimately deliver better outcomes for individuals affected by this common skin cancer. In this chapter, we will delve into the emerging technologies, innovations, and research priorities that are shaping the future of basal cell carcinoma care.

Emerging Technologies and Innovations

The field of basal cell carcinoma management has witnessed a steady stream of technological advancements and innovative approaches, each with the potential to revolutionize the way we detect, treat, and monitor this prevalent skin malignancy.

Advancements in Imaging Techniques

The continuous development and refinement of imaging technologies have significantly enhanced the diagnostic capabilities for basal cell carcinoma, enabling healthcare providers to visualize and characterize these lesions with greater precision.

1. High-resolution optical coherence tomography (HR-OCT): This non-invasive, high-resolution imaging technique can provide detailed, cross-sectional visualization of the skin's microstructure, allowing for the identification of characteristic features associated with BCC, such as the depth of tumor invasion and the presence of subclinical extensions.

2. Artificial intelligence (AI)-assisted dermoscopy: The integration of machine learning algorithms into the analysis of dermoscopic images can assist healthcare providers in the accurate detection and classification of basal cell carcinoma lesions, potentially improving diagnostic accuracy and reducing variability among clinicians.

3. Fluorescence imaging: Emerging fluorescence-based imaging techniques, such as confocal fluorescence microscopy, can leverage the selective accumulation of fluorescent probes within BCC tumor cells, enabling the real-time visualization and delineation of lesion borders during surgical procedures.

These advancements in imaging modalities not only improve diagnostic accuracy but also have the potential to guide more tailored treatment approaches, optimize surgical planning, and enhance the monitoring of treatment response and disease recurrence.

Advancements in Genomic and Molecular Profiling

The growing understanding of the genetic and molecular underpinnings of basal cell carcinoma has paved the way for the development of innovative diagnostic and predictive tools, as well as the exploration of personalized, targeted therapies.

1. Genomic profiling: The comprehensive analysis of the genetic alterations within BCC tumors, using techniques such as next-generation sequencing, can provide valuable insights into the molecular drivers of the disease, potentially identifying novel therapeutic targets and guiding the selection of

targeted treatments.

2. Biomarker-driven diagnostics: The identification of specific molecular biomarkers associated with basal cell carcinoma, such as mutations in the PTCH1 and SMO genes, can facilitate the development of highly sensitive and specific diagnostic tests, enabling earlier detection and more personalized management approaches.

3. Liquid biopsy: The analysis of circulating tumor cells or cell-free tumor DNA in the blood, known as liquid biopsy, can provide a non-invasive approach to monitor disease status, detect recurrence, and potentially guide the selection of targeted therapies for advanced or metastatic BCC cases.

These advancements in genomic and molecular profiling have the potential to transform the way healthcare providers approach the diagnosis, risk stratification, and treatment selection for patients with basal cell carcinoma, ultimately leading to more personalized and effective care.

Innovations in Therapeutic Modalities

In addition to the improvements in diagnostic capabilities, the field of basal cell carcinoma management is also witnessing the emergence of novel therapeutic approaches, offering new avenues for the treatment of this common skin cancer.

1. Targeted drug delivery systems: The development of specialized drug delivery systems, such as nanoparticle-based formulations or microneedle patches, can enhance the targeted delivery of therapeutic agents to BCC lesions, potentially improving treatment efficacy and reducing systemic toxicity.

2. Immunotherapeutic approaches: The exploration of immunotherapeutic strategies, including the use of immune checkpoint inhibitors or oncolytic

viruses, aims to harness the body's own immune system to recognize and eliminate basal cell carcinoma tumor cells.

3. Regenerative medicine and tissue engineering: Innovative approaches in the field of regenerative medicine, such as the use of stem cell-based therapies or tissue-engineered skin substitutes, may provide new avenues for the reconstruction and regeneration of tissue after the surgical removal of BCC lesions, ultimately improving cosmetic and functional outcomes.

4. Combination therapies: The integration of various treatment modalities, including targeted systemic therapies, topical agents, and radiation therapy, may offer synergistic effects and improve clinical outcomes for patients with advanced or high-risk basal cell carcinoma.

These emerging therapeutic innovations hold the promise of expanding the treatment options, enhancing the efficacy, and improving the safety and tolerability of BCC management, ultimately leading to better overall outcomes for individuals affected by this common skin cancer.

Clinical Trials and Ongoing Studies

The pursuit of improved basal cell carcinoma management is fueled by a robust pipeline of clinical trials and ongoing research studies, exploring a wide range of novel diagnostic approaches, therapeutic interventions, and disease prevention strategies.

Investigational Diagnostic Techniques

Clinical trials are currently evaluating the use of various advanced imaging modalities, such as high-resolution optical coherence tomography and artificial intelligence-assisted dermoscopy, to enhance the accuracy and efficiency of BCC detection and characterization.

Additionally, studies are investigating the potential utility of molecular biomarkers and liquid biopsy techniques in the early diagnosis, risk stratification, and disease monitoring of basal cell carcinoma.

Emerging Therapeutic Interventions

The clinical research landscape for basal cell carcinoma management is particularly dynamic, with a focus on the development and evaluation of innovative therapeutic approaches, including:

1. Novel targeted therapies: Clinical trials are exploring the efficacy and safety of next-generation Hedgehog pathway inhibitors, as well as investigating the potential of other targeted agents that may disrupt critical signaling cascades involved in BCC pathogenesis.

2. Immunotherapeutic strategies: Researchers are evaluating the use of immune checkpoint inhibitors, oncolytic viruses, and other immunotherapeutic approaches, either as monotherapies or in combination with conventional treatments, for the management of advanced or metastatic basal cell carcinoma.

3. Combination treatment regimens: Clinical studies are investigating the synergistic effects of combining various treatment modalities, such as topical agents, radiation therapy, and systemic therapies, to improve outcomes for patients with high-risk or recurrent BCC lesions.

4. Regenerative and tissue engineering approaches: Investigational studies are exploring the potential of stem cell-based therapies and engineered skin substitutes to enhance tissue regeneration and improve cosmetic and functional outcomes after the surgical treatment of basal cell carcinoma.

Prevention and Risk Reduction Strategies

In addition to the focus on diagnostic and therapeutic innovations, clinical research is also exploring strategies for the prevention and risk reduction of basal cell carcinoma.

Areas of investigation include:

1. Chemoprevention: Clinical trials are evaluating the use of topical or systemic agents, such as retinoids or nonsteroidal anti-inflammatory drugs (NSAIDs), for their potential to prevent the development or recurrence of BCC lesions.

2. Lifestyle and behavioral interventions: Studies are examining the impact of dietary modifications, sun protection measures, and other lifestyle factors on the risk of basal cell carcinoma, with the aim of developing evidence-based prevention strategies.

3. Genetic and biomarker-guided risk assessment: Researchers are exploring the use of genetic and molecular profiling to identify individuals at a higher risk of developing BCC, enabling the implementation of personalized prevention and screening protocols.

By actively participating in and supporting these clinical trials and ongoing research initiatives, healthcare providers can stay at the forefront of the latest advancements in basal cell carcinoma management, ensuring that their patients have access to the most promising diagnostic and therapeutic options.

Personalized Medicine and Targeted Therapies

The growing understanding of the genetic and molecular underpinnings of basal cell carcinoma has paved the way for the emergence of personalized medicine and targeted therapies, transforming the way healthcare providers approach the management of this common skin cancer.

Genetic and Molecular Profiling

The comprehensive genomic and molecular characterization of basal cell carcinoma tumors has revealed a wealth of information about the key genetic alterations and signaling pathways that drive the development and progression of this disease.

By leveraging this knowledge, healthcare providers can:

1. Identify individuals with a heightened genetic predisposition to BCC, enabling the implementation of personalized prevention and early detection strategies.
2. Analyze the specific genetic and molecular profiles of individual BCC lesions, guiding the selection of the most appropriate targeted therapies and tailoring the management approach to the unique characteristics of the tumor.
3. Monitor for the emergence of drug resistance mechanisms and guide the selection of alternative or combination treatment strategies to overcome these challenges.

Targeted Therapies and Combination Approaches

The advancement in the understanding of BCC's genetic and molecular underpinnings has led to the development of highly targeted therapeutic agents, such as Hedgehog pathway inhibitors, which have revolutionized the management of advanced and metastatic basal cell carcinoma.

Furthermore, the integration of these targeted therapies with other treatment modalities, including surgical interventions, radiation therapy, and immunotherapies, has the potential to optimize treatment outcomes and minimize the risk of disease recurrence or progression.

As the field of personalized medicine continues to evolve, healthcare providers will increasingly be able to leverage genetic and molecular profiling to deliver truly individualized care, tailoring the diagnostic, preventive, and therapeutic approaches to the unique needs and characteristics of each patient with basal cell carcinoma.

Optimizing Patient Outcomes and Quality of Life

Alongside the technological and scientific advancements in basal cell carcinoma management, the future of this field must also prioritize the optimization of patient outcomes and quality of life. This holistic, patient-centered approach will be critical in ensuring that individuals affected by this common skin cancer receive comprehensive, high-quality care that addresses their multifaceted needs.

Enhancing Patient-Reported Outcomes

The systematic collection and analysis of patient-reported outcome measures (PROMs) will play a pivotal role in evaluating the impact of BCC management on the patient's overall well-being, including their physical, emotional, and functional outcomes.

By incorporating PROMs into clinical practice and research, healthcare providers can:

1. Gain valuable insights into the patient's experience and the factors that are most important to them, such as cosmetic outcomes, symptom burden, and quality of life.
2. Utilize this patient-centered data to guide the selection of treatment approaches, optimize shared decision-making, and tailor the care plan to the individual's preferences and needs.
3. Monitor the long-term impact of BCC management on the patient's

overall health and well-being, enabling the continuous improvement of care delivery.

Integrating Digital Health Technologies

The integration of digital health technologies, such as mobile applications, wearable devices, and telehealth platforms, can significantly enhance patient engagement, improve access to care, and enable more personalized, data-driven management of basal cell carcinoma.

These digital health tools can:

1. Facilitate remote monitoring of BCC lesions, enabling early detection of recurrence or new lesions and promoting timely intervention.
2. Empower patients to actively participate in their skin self-examination, skin cancer prevention, and long-term follow-up care.
3. Improve access to specialized dermatological services for individuals in underserved or geographically remote areas, reducing barriers to care.
4. Foster better communication and collaboration between patients and their healthcare providers, enhancing the coordination and continuity of BCC management.

By embracing these patient-centered innovations and digital health technologies, the future of basal cell carcinoma care will be increasingly focused on delivering personalized, high-quality services that optimize outcomes and enhance the overall quality of life for individuals affected by this common skin cancer.

Conclusion

The future of basal cell carcinoma management is marked by a dynamic landscape of technological advancements, innovative therapeutic approaches, and a growing emphasis on personalized, patient-centered care. The continued exploration of emerging imaging modalities, genomic and molecular profiling techniques, and novel therapeutic interventions holds the promise of enhancing diagnostic capabilities, improving treatment outcomes, and ultimately reducing the burden of this prevalent skin malignancy.

As the field of BCC management evolves, healthcare providers must remain vigilant in staying abreast of the latest research, best practices, and evidence-based guidelines to ensure that their patients receive the most comprehensive and cutting-edge care. By integrating these innovations into their clinical practice and collaborating with researchers and policymakers, healthcare providers can play a pivotal role in shaping the future of basal cell carcinoma management and improving the overall well-being of individuals affected by this condition.

The insights and vision outlined in this chapter will serve as a foundation for the final chapter, which will focus on the critical role of patient empowerment, education, and the importance of navigating the healthcare system in the comprehensive management of basal cell carcinoma.

CHAPTER 13

C hapter 13: Patient Empowerment and Education

In the comprehensive management of basal cell carcinoma (BCC), the active engagement and empowerment of patients are essential components for achieving optimal outcomes. By equipping individuals with a deep understanding of their condition, the available treatment options, and the resources to navigate the healthcare system, healthcare providers can empower patients to become active participants in their own care, leading to improved adherence, better-informed decision-making, and ultimately, enhanced overall well-being.

In this chapter, we will explore strategies for patient empowerment and education, highlighting the critical role of patient-provider communication, the importance of accessible information resources, and the significance of navigating the healthcare system in the comprehensive management of basal cell carcinoma.

Understanding the Disease and Treatment Options

The foundation of patient empowerment begins with a comprehensive understanding of basal cell carcinoma, its characteristics, and the available management strategies. Healthcare providers must prioritize the education of their patients, ensuring they have the necessary knowledge to actively participate in their care.

Educating Patients about Basal Cell Carcinoma

Patients should be provided with clear and concise information about the following aspects of basal cell carcinoma:

1. Definition and classification: Explaining the nature of BCC as a common type of skin cancer and the various subtypes (e.g., nodular, infiltrative, superficial) can help patients understand the complexity of the disease.

2. Risk factors and causes: Educating patients about the role of UV exposure, genetic factors, and other contributory elements can empower them to take proactive steps towards prevention and early detection.

3. Diagnostic process: Outlining the diagnostic tools, such as visual examination, dermatoscopy, and biopsy, can prepare patients for the evaluation of any suspicious skin lesions.

4. Prognosis and outcomes: Providing realistic information about the generally favorable prognosis of BCC, as well as the potential for recurrence or advanced disease, can help manage patient expectations and promote shared decision-making.

By fostering a comprehensive understanding of basal cell carcinoma, healthcare providers can enable patients to make informed choices and actively participate in their care.

Communicating Treatment Options

Equally important is the patient's understanding of the available treatment options for basal cell carcinoma, including both surgical and non-surgical approaches. Healthcare providers should:

1. Explain the various treatment modalities, such as surgical excision, Mohs micrographic surgery, topical medications, and radiation therapy, in a clear and accessible manner.
2. Discuss the potential benefits, risks, and expected outcomes associated with each treatment option, empowering patients to weigh the pros and cons and make informed decisions.
3. Encourage patients to ask questions, express their preferences, and voice any concerns they may have about the proposed treatment plan.

This open and transparent communication helps to establish a collaborative partnership between the healthcare provider and the patient, fostering a shared decision-making process that aligns with the patient's individual goals, values, and needs.

Navigating the Healthcare System

Basal cell carcinoma management often involves navigating a complex healthcare system, which can be challenging for patients. Healthcare providers play a crucial role in guiding patients through this process, ensuring they have the necessary knowledge and resources to access the appropriate care.

Guidance on Healthcare Utilization

Healthcare providers should educate patients on the various components of the healthcare system, including:

1. Identifying the appropriate healthcare providers (e.g., dermatologists, primary care physicians, Mohs surgeons) and their respective roles in BCC management.
2. Explaining the importance of regular skin cancer screenings, follow-up

visits, and the coordination of care among different specialists.

3. Providing information on insurance coverage, payment options, and financial assistance programs that may be available to support the cost of BCC diagnosis and treatment.

By empowering patients with this knowledge, healthcare providers can help them navigate the healthcare system more effectively, reducing barriers to care and ensuring timely access to the necessary services.

Facilitating Coordinated Care

The management of basal cell carcinoma often requires the involvement of multiple healthcare providers, including dermatologists, oncologists, radiation oncologists, and plastic surgeons. Healthcare providers should:

1. Facilitate the coordination of care among the various specialists involved in the patient's treatment plan, ensuring seamless communication and the alignment of the overall management approach.
2. Provide patients with clear information about the roles and responsibilities of each healthcare provider, as well as their contact information, to promote effective communication and collaboration.
3. Assist patients in scheduling appointments, arranging referrals, and navigating the transitions between different healthcare settings, helping to minimize the burden on the patient.

By promoting a coordinated, patient-centered approach to care, healthcare providers can empower patients to actively participate in the management of their basal cell carcinoma, leading to improved outcomes and overall satisfaction with the healthcare experience.

Patient Support and Resources

In addition to providing comprehensive education and guidance on navigating the healthcare system, healthcare providers should also connect patients with relevant support resources and tools to enhance their overall management of basal cell carcinoma.

Patient Education Materials

Developing and providing patients with easy-to-understand educational materials, such as brochures, website resources, or multimedia content, can reinforce the information shared during clinical encounters and serve as a valuable reference for patients.

These educational resources should cover topics such as:

1. BCC risk factors and prevention strategies
2. Self-examination techniques and the importance of early detection
3. Detailed explanations of the various treatment options
4. Guidance on managing treatment-related side effects and complications
5. Information on long-term follow-up care and skin cancer survivorship

By making these resources readily available and accessible, healthcare providers can empower patients to take an active role in their care and refer back to the information as needed.

Patient Support Groups and Networks

Connecting patients with support groups, either in-person or online, can provide a valuable source of emotional, informational, and social support. These peer-to-peer networks can help patients:

1. Share their experiences, coping strategies, and insights with others facing similar challenges.
2. Learn from the experiences of other patients and caregivers, gaining valuable practical advice.
3. Feel less isolated and more connected to a community of individuals affected by basal cell carcinoma.

Healthcare providers can facilitate these connections by providing patients with referrals to reputable patient advocacy organizations or by facilitating the establishment of local support groups within their healthcare settings.

Cultivating a Culture of Patient Empowerment

To truly foster a comprehensive approach to patient empowerment in the management of basal cell carcinoma, healthcare providers must work towards cultivating a culture of patient-centered care within their healthcare settings.

Promoting Shared Decision-Making

Shared decision-making is a fundamental aspect of patient empowerment, where healthcare providers and patients collaborate to make informed choices about the management of the patient's condition. This approach involves:

1. Eliciting the patient's preferences, values, and goals for their care.
2. Providing the patient with comprehensive, evidence-based information about the available treatment options and their potential benefits and risks.
3. Engaging the patient in the decision-making process and incorporating their input into the final treatment plan.

By embracing shared decision-making, healthcare providers can empower patients to take an active role in their care, leading to better alignment between the treatment approach and the individual's needs and priorities.

Encouraging Patient Feedback and Engagement

Healthcare providers should actively seek and incorporate patient feedback to continuously improve the delivery of care and enhance the patient experience. This may include:

1. Regularly collecting and analyzing patient-reported outcome measures (PROMs) to assess the impact of BCC management on the patient's quality of life and overall well-being.
2. Soliciting patient feedback through surveys, focus groups, or patient advisory councils to identify areas for improvement and implement patient-centered initiatives.
3. Fostering a culture of open communication, where patients feel comfortable voicing their concerns, questions, or suggestions to their healthcare providers.

By actively engaging patients and responding to their feedback, healthcare providers can demonstrate their commitment to patient empowerment and continuously strive to deliver care that aligns with the unique needs and preferences of individuals affected by basal cell carcinoma.

Collaborating with Patient Advocacy Organizations

Partnering with patient advocacy organizations can be a valuable strategy for healthcare providers to amplify the voices of patients, access educational resources, and collaborate on initiatives that promote patient empowerment.

These organizations can serve as:

1. Trusted sources of information and support for patients and their families.
2. Advocates for improved access to care, research funding, and the development of patient-centered policies.
3. Collaborative partners in the design and implementation of educational campaigns, awareness programs, and patient-focused initiatives.

By fostering these partnerships, healthcare providers can leverage the expertise and reach of patient advocacy groups to empower their patients and enhance the overall management of basal cell carcinoma.

Conclusion

Patient empowerment and education are essential components in the comprehensive management of basal cell carcinoma. By equipping patients with a deep understanding of their condition, the available treatment options, and the resources to navigate the healthcare system, healthcare providers can empower individuals to become active participants in their own care, leading to improved outcomes, better-informed decision-making, and enhanced overall well-being.

Through effective communication, the provision of accessible educational resources, and the facilitation of coordinated care, healthcare providers can foster a culture of patient-centered care that prioritizes shared decision-making, patient feedback, and collaborative partnerships with patient advocacy organizations.

By embracing this holistic, patient-empowered approach to basal cell carcinoma management, healthcare providers can ensure that individuals affected by this common skin cancer receive the comprehensive, personalized care they deserve, ultimately improving their quality of life and reducing the burden of this condition.

The insights and strategies discussed in this chapter serve as a culmination of the comprehensive knowledge and best practices outlined throughout this book, highlighting the critical role of patient engagement and education in the overall management of basal cell carcinoma.

CHAPTER 14

C hapter 14: Conclusion and Key Takeaways

As we reach the culmination of this comprehensive exploration of basal cell carcinoma (BCC), it is essential to synthesize the key insights, best practices, and takeaways that have been discussed throughout this book. The management of basal cell carcinoma is a complex and multifaceted endeavor, requiring healthcare providers to navigate a vast array of considerations, from understanding the fundamental aspects of the disease to implementing innovative and personalized treatment approaches.

In this final chapter, we will distill the most salient points and highlight the overarching principles that should guide the comprehensive care of individuals affected by basal cell carcinoma, empowering healthcare providers to deliver the highest standard of care and ultimately improve patient outcomes and quality of life.

Summary of Best Practices and Guidelines

Basal cell carcinoma is a prevalent skin cancer that requires a thorough understanding of its definition, classification, epidemiology, and underlying pathophysiology. Healthcare providers must be equipped with the knowledge to accurately diagnose BCC, differentiate its diverse subtypes, and recognize the key risk factors that contribute to its development.

Early detection and prevention are cornerstones of effective BCC management. Empowering patients to perform regular skin self-examinations, incorporating routine skin cancer screening into primary care, and implementing targeted risk stratification strategies are crucial for identifying BCC lesions at their earliest stages, when treatment is most effective and the potential for favorable outcomes is highest.

The selection of the appropriate treatment approach, whether it be surgical interventions, non-surgical modalities, or a combination thereof, must be guided by a comprehensive assessment of the BCC lesion's characteristics, the patient's individual factors and preferences, and the expertise and resources available within the healthcare setting. Healthcare providers must prioritize the balance between complete tumor removal, the preservation of healthy tissue, and the optimization of cosmetic and functional outcomes.

For advanced and metastatic BCC cases, a multidisciplinary, collaborative approach is essential, leveraging the expertise of specialists in dermatology, oncology, radiation oncology, and plastic surgery. The integration of targeted systemic therapies, such as Hedgehog pathway inhibitors, has revolutionized the management of these high-risk cases, offering new hope and improved outcomes for affected individuals.

Across the spectrum of BCC management, the importance of long-term follow-up, skin cancer prevention strategies, and the provision of psychological and emotional support cannot be overstated. Comprehensive survivorship care planning, the cultivation of patient resilience, and the incorporation of integrative and complementary approaches are all crucial components of delivering holistic, patient-centered care.

Underlying these best practices and guidelines is the recognition that basal cell carcinoma management must be tailored to the unique needs and circumstances of each individual patient. Healthcare providers must embrace a shared decision-making approach, empowering patients to be active participants in their care and ensuring that the selected interventions align with the patient's values, preferences, and overall well-being.

Optimizing Basal Cell Carcinoma Management

The comprehensive management of basal cell carcinoma requires healthcare providers to adopt a multifaceted, evidence-based approach that addresses the diverse aspects of this prevalent skin cancer. By synthesizing the key insights and best practices discussed throughout this book, several overarching principles emerge as essential for optimizing the care of individuals affected by BCC:

1. Comprehensive understanding of the disease: Healthcare providers must possess a thorough understanding of the fundamental aspects of basal cell carcinoma, including its definition, classification, epidemiology, and underlying pathophysiology, to inform accurate diagnosis and appropriate management strategies.

2. Early detection and prevention: Prioritizing the implementation of effective screening, risk stratification, and patient education strategies is crucial for identifying BCC lesions at their earliest stages, when treatment is most effective and the potential for favorable outcomes is highest.

3. Personalized, multidisciplinary care: The selection and integration of treatment modalities, whether surgical, non-surgical, or a combination thereof, must be tailored to the unique characteristics of the BCC lesion and the individual patient's needs, preferences, and overall health status. This often requires the collaboration of a multidisciplinary team of healthcare providers to deliver comprehensive, patient-centered care.

4. Innovative and evidence-based approaches: Healthcare providers must remain vigilant in staying abreast of the latest advancements, emerging technologies, and evidence-based guidelines in the field of basal cell carcinoma

management, ensuring that their patients have access to the most promising diagnostic and therapeutic options.

5. Emphasis on quality of life and patient empowerment: The management of basal cell carcinoma must extend beyond the mere treatment of the tumor, prioritizing the optimization of cosmetic and functional outcomes, the provision of psychological and emotional support, and the empowerment of patients to become active participants in their own care.

6. Addressing health disparities and global perspectives: Recognizing and addressing the geographic, socioeconomic, and demographic disparities that impact the incidence, management, and outcomes of basal cell carcinoma is crucial for promoting equitable access to high-quality care and improving overall disease burden worldwide.

7. Continuous learning and collaboration: Healthcare providers must foster a culture of continuous learning, actively engaging in research, clinical trials, and interdisciplinary collaborations to advance the understanding and management of basal cell carcinoma, ultimately leading to improved patient outcomes and the reduction of the overall burden of this prevalent skin cancer.

By embracing these overarching principles and integrating the comprehensive best practices and guidelines outlined throughout this book, healthcare providers can deliver the highest standard of care for individuals affected by basal cell carcinoma, ensuring that their patients receive personalized, evidence-based, and patient-centered management that optimizes their overall well-being and quality of life.

Improving Patient Outcomes and Quality of Life

At the heart of the comprehensive management of basal cell carcinoma lies the unwavering commitment to improving patient outcomes and enhancing the overall quality of life for individuals affected by this condition. This patient-centered approach should be the driving force behind the continued evolution and optimization of BCC care.

Through the implementation of effective prevention strategies, early detection techniques, and personalized treatment approaches, healthcare providers can work towards achieving the following key objectives:

1. Reducing the incidence and burden of basal cell carcinoma: By empowering patients to adopt sun-safe behaviors, prioritizing routine skin cancer screening, and addressing health disparities, the overall incidence and burden of BCC can be reduced, leading to improved population-level outcomes.

2. Enhancing disease control and minimizing recurrence: The utilization of evidence-based diagnostic tools and the selection of appropriate treatment modalities, tailored to the specific characteristics of the BCC lesion, can help achieve complete tumor removal and minimize the risk of local recurrence or the development of new primary tumors.

3. Optimizing cosmetic and functional outcomes: Prioritizing the preservation of healthy tissue, employing specialized surgical and reconstructive techniques, and addressing the psychological and emotional impact of BCC can lead to improved aesthetic and functional outcomes, positively impacting the patient's overall quality of life.

4. Improving long-term survivorship and quality of life: Comprehensive survivorship care, including regular monitoring for recurrence, skin cancer prevention strategies, and the provision of psychological and emotional support, can help BCC survivors maintain their skin health, manage the long-term effects of the disease, and thrive in their daily lives.

5. Empowering patients to be active participants in their care: By fostering a culture of patient empowerment, healthcare providers can enable individuals

affected by basal cell carcinoma to make informed decisions, actively engage in their own care, and ultimately achieve better outcomes and a greater sense of control over their health.

Through the collective efforts of healthcare providers, researchers, policy-makers, and patient advocacy organizations, the continued pursuit of these patient-centric objectives will undoubtedly lead to the enhancement of basal cell carcinoma management and the improvement of overall outcomes and quality of life for all individuals affected by this prevalent skin malignancy.

Conclusion

The comprehensive management of basal cell carcinoma is a multifaceted and ever-evolving endeavor, requiring healthcare providers to possess a deep understanding of the disease, adopt evidence-based best practices, and embrace a patient-centered approach that prioritizes the optimization of outcomes and the enhancement of quality of life.

By synthesizing the key insights and strategies discussed throughout this book, several overarching principles emerge as essential for the delivery of high-quality, comprehensive BCC care. These principles include the impor-tance of a thorough understanding of the disease, the prioritization of early detection and prevention, the adoption of personalized, multidisciplinary approaches, the integration of innovative and evidence-based interventions, the emphasis on quality of life and patient empowerment, the recognition and mitigation of health disparities, and the cultivation of a culture of continuous learning and collaboration.

Ultimately, the successful management of basal cell carcinoma hinges on the unwavering commitment of healthcare providers to improve patient outcomes and enhance the overall quality of life for individuals affected by this prevalent skin cancer. Through the implementation of effective prevention strategies, the utilization of cutting-edge diagnostic and treatment modalities, and the delivery of comprehensive, patient-centered care, healthcare providers can work towards reducing the burden of basal cell carcinoma and ensuring that all patients receive the high-quality, personalized management they deserve.

As the field of basal cell carcinoma management continues to evolve, healthcare providers must remain vigilant, stay at the forefront of the latest advancements, and embrace a holistic, collaborative approach to care. By doing so, they can contribute to the ongoing efforts to conquer the challenge of basal cell carcinoma and improve the lives of those affected by this common, yet complex, skin malignancy.

CONCLUSION

Conquering the Challenge of Basal Cell Carcinoma: A Comprehensive Approach to Improved Outcomes and Enhanced Quality of Life

As we reach the culmination of this comprehensive exploration of basal cell carcinoma (BCC), it is essential to reflect on the overarching principles and key takeaways that have been woven throughout the chapters of this book. The management of basal cell carcinoma is a multifaceted and ever-evolving endeavor, requiring healthcare providers to navigate a complex landscape of clinical considerations, emerging technologies, and patient-centered care.

At the heart of this comprehensive approach to basal cell carcinoma lies the unwavering commitment to improving patient outcomes and enhancing the overall quality of life for individuals affected by this prevalent skin cancer. Through the collective efforts of healthcare providers, researchers, policymakers, and patient advocacy organizations, significant strides have been made in the understanding, prevention, and management of BCC. However, the work is far from over, as we continue to face new challenges and seek innovative solutions to conquer this common, yet complex, skin malignancy.

The Foundations of Comprehensive BCC Management

The foundation of effective basal cell carcinoma management begins with a thorough understanding of the disease itself. Healthcare providers must possess a deep knowledge of BCC's definition, classification, epidemiology, and underlying pathophysiology to accurately diagnose, risk-stratify, and implement appropriate management strategies for their patients.

Equally crucial is the prioritization of early detection and prevention. By empowering patients to perform regular skin self-examinations, incorporating routine skin cancer screening into primary care, and implementing targeted risk stratification approaches, healthcare providers can identify BCC lesions at their earliest stages, when treatment is most effective and the potential for favorable outcomes is highest.

The selection of the appropriate treatment modality, whether it be surgical interventions, non-surgical approaches, or a combination thereof, must be guided by a comprehensive assessment of the BCC lesion's characteristics, the patient's individual factors and preferences, and the expertise and resources available within the healthcare setting. This personalized, multidisciplinary approach to care is essential for optimizing treatment outcomes and minimizing the impact on the patient's quality of life.

Advancements and Innovations in BCC Management

The field of basal cell carcinoma management has witnessed a steady stream of technological advancements and innovative approaches, each with the potential to revolutionize the way we detect, treat, and monitor this prevalent skin cancer.

From the integration of cutting-edge imaging techniques, such as high-resolution optical coherence tomography and artificial intelligence-assisted dermoscopy, to the exploration of personalized, targeted therapies that leverage the genetic and molecular underpinnings of BCC, the healthcare landscape is continuously evolving. These innovations hold the promise of enhancing diagnostic capabilities, improving treatment efficacy, and ultimately delivering better outcomes for individuals affected by basal cell carcinoma.

Furthermore, the ongoing exploration of novel therapeutic interventions, including immunotherapeutic strategies, regenerative medicine approaches, and the integration of combination treatment regimens, offers new avenues for the management of advanced, recurrent, or high-risk BCC cases. As these investigational modalities advance through clinical trials and become integrated into standard practice, healthcare providers will have an expanded arsenal of tools to tackle the complexities of basal cell carcinoma.

Embracing a Patient-Centered Approach

While the advancements in diagnostic techniques and therapeutic options are undoubtedly important, the comprehensive management of basal cell carcinoma must also prioritize the optimization of patient outcomes and the enhancement of quality of life. This patient-centered approach is essential for ensuring that individuals affected by BCC receive care that addresses their multifaceted needs, from the physical to the psychological and emotional.

Empowering patients to become active participants in their own care, through effective communication, the provision of accessible educational resources, and the facilitation of coordinated care, is a crucial component of this patient-centered model. By fostering a culture of shared decision-making, healthcare providers can align the management plan with the patient's values, preferences, and overall well-being, ultimately leading to better adherence, improved outcomes, and a greater sense of control over the disease.

Furthermore, the recognition and mitigation of health disparities in basal cell carcinoma care are essential for promoting equity and ensuring that all individuals, regardless of their geographic location, socioeconomic status, or demographic background, have access to high-quality, evidence-based management. By addressing these systemic barriers and fostering global collaborations, healthcare providers and policymakers can work towards reducing the overall burden of BCC and improving outcomes for diverse populations worldwide.

Navigating the Future of Basal Cell Carcinoma Management

As we look towards the future of basal cell carcinoma management, the path forward is marked by a continued commitment to innovation, collaboration, and a steadfast focus on improving patient outcomes and quality of life.

Healthcare providers must remain vigilant in staying abreast of the latest advancements, emerging technologies, and evidence-based guidelines in the field of BCC care. By embracing a culture of continuous learning and actively engaging in research, clinical trials, and interdisciplinary collaborations, they can contribute to the advancement of this field and ensure that their patients have access to the most promising diagnostic and therapeutic options.

Additionally, the integration of patient-centered initiatives, such as the systematic collection and analysis of patient-reported outcome measures, the utilization of digital health technologies, and the fostering of partnerships with patient advocacy organizations, will be crucial in delivering truly comprehensive, personalized care that addresses the holistic needs of individuals affected by basal cell carcinoma.

Ultimately, the future of basal cell carcinoma management must be guided by a relentless pursuit of improved outcomes and enhanced quality of life for all patients. Through the collective efforts of healthcare providers, researchers, policymakers, and patient advocates, we can work towards the shared goal of conquering the challenge of this prevalent skin cancer and ensuring that every individual affected by BCC receives the high-quality, personalized care they deserve.

Embracing the Call to Action

As we conclude this comprehensive exploration of basal cell carcinoma, the call to action is clear: healthcare providers, researchers, and policymakers must come together to elevate the standard of care, address the global disparities, and empower patients to take an active role in the management of this common skin cancer.

By embracing the overarching principles and key takeaways outlined throughout this book, healthcare providers can deliver the highest quality of care, optimize patient outcomes, and enhance the overall well-being of individuals affected by basal cell carcinoma. These principles include:

1. Maintaining a comprehensive understanding of the disease and its underlying mechanisms
2. Prioritizing early detection and prevention through effective screening and patient education
3. Adopting personalized, multidisciplinary approaches to treatment selection and management
4. Integrating innovative, evidence-based interventions to enhance diagnostic capabilities and improve therapeutic options
5. Prioritizing the optimization of quality of life and the empowerment of patients as active participants in their care
6. Addressing health disparities and fostering global collaborations to promote equitable access to high-quality BCC management
7. Cultivating a culture of continuous learning, research, and interdisciplinary collaboration to advance the field

By steadfastly adhering to these guiding principles, healthcare providers can ensure that the care they deliver for individuals affected by basal cell carcinoma is comprehensive, patient-centered, and optimized for the best possible outcomes.

Furthermore, the call to action extends beyond the healthcare community, encompassing the roles of researchers, policymakers, and patient advocacy organizations. Continued investment in BCC-related research, the development of evidence-based guidelines and policies, and the amplification of patient voices are all crucial components in the collective effort to conquer this prevalent skin cancer.

As we look to the future, the path forward is clear: through the unwavering commitment to innovation, collaboration, and a steadfast focus on improving patient outcomes and quality of life, we can make significant strides in the management of basal cell carcinoma. By embracing this call to action, we can work together to reduce the burden of this disease, enhance the well-being of those affected, and ultimately, conquer the challenge of basal cell carcinoma.